Gendered Moods

Tranquillisers are prescribed twice as often to women as men, yet little gender-based research has been carried out on the social context of their use.

Gendered Moods offers the first feminist analysis of the gendered character of psychotropic drug use, based on studies of long-term psychotropic drug users and the content of drug advertising. The authors argue that gender differences in psychotropic drug use are manifestations of the gendered construction of society as a whole, and that, as a result, women are particularly susceptible to being channelled into a state of dependency on prescribed drugs.

Exploring current social scientific debates relating to drug users and providers, *Gendered Moods* also provides a critical review of previous research, and concludes that gender has been underestimated as an influence on the use and effects of these drugs. It will give a much needed introduction to a neglected area of study.

Elizabeth Ettorre is Docent in Sociology at Åbo Akademi University and the University of Helsinki, Finland, and the author of *Lesbians, Women and Society* and *Women and Substance Abuse*. **Elianne Riska** is Professor of Sociology at Åbo Akademi University, Åbo, Finland, and the author of *Power, Politics and Health: Forces Shaping American Medicine* and *Gender, Work and Medicine*.

Gendered Moods

Psychotropics and society

Elizabeth Ettorre and
Elianne Riska

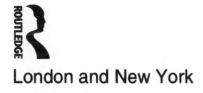

London and New York

First published 1995
by Routledge
2 Park Square, Milton Park, Abingdon,Oxon, OX14 4RN
Simultaneously published in the USA and Canada
by Routledge
711 Third Avenue, New York, NY 10017

© 1995 Elizabeth Ettorre and Elianne Riska

Typeset in Palatino by LaserScript, Mitcham, Surrey

British Library Cataloguing in Publication Data
A catalogue record for this book is available from the British Library

Library of Congress Cataloguing in Publication Data
A catalogue record for this book has been requested

ISBN 0–415–08213–7 (hbk)
ISBN 0–415–08214–5 (pbk)

Contents

Contents

Tables

Acknowledgements

This book is the result of our collaborative work as feminist scholars and women sociologists, working in the field of medical and health sociology and women's studies. There are many who have provided support in making this book possible. First, we would like to thank Heather Gibson, our editor at Routledge, who invited us to do this book and who has been consistently patient and supportive of our endeavour. We are also grateful to the Medical Research Council of the Academy of Finland which provided funding for our research project, 'The social meaning of psychotropic drug use: developing a gender-sensitive perspective', from August 1991 until July 1992. Many ideas for this book have been based on our study. Timo Klaukka from the National Institute for Social Security, Social Insurance Institution, Helsinki, Finland, has provided continual information and advice on the medical and pharmacological aspects of psychotropics throughout our study and during the writing of this book. We owe him a special vote of thanks.

Our colleagues from the Department of Sociology and the Institute of Women's Studies at Åbo Akademi University have also provided much needed support, collegial advice and practical assistance: Johanna Österberg, Maria Grönroos and Ulrica Hägglund. Karin Kvideland deserves special thanks for her help and patience, particularly during the final stages of the writing process.

This work has also been influenced by our fruitful discussions over the years with both American and British colleagues who have helped us to explore a variety of important theoretical issues. Of course, we are most grateful to our nearest and dearest for their support and encouragement.

Some of the ideas presented in Chapters 1 and 2 as well as some data provided in Chapters 6, 7 and 8 appeared originally in article form and have been elaborated upon in this book: E. Ettorre and E. Riska (1993) 'Psychotropics, sociology and women: are the "halcyon" days of the malestream over?', *Sociology of Health and Illness* 15: 503–24; and E. Ettorre, T. Klaukka and E. Riska (1994) 'Psychotropic drugs: long-term use, dependency and the gender factor', *Social Science and Medicine* 39, 12: 1667–73.

Elizabeth Ettorre and Elianne Riska

Chapter 1

Introduction
Psychotropics and women – setting the scene

WHAT ARE PSYCHOTROPICS?

Anxiety and sleeplessness are in the popular culture referred to as 'stress', a concept which denotes both the stressful circumstances of life and the concomitant experience of symptoms. A pharmacological way to deal with stress symptoms and uncomfortable moods has been developed in modern society: a drug group, called tranquillisers. Tranquillisers, such as Valium, Librium, Halcion, Ativan, to name a few, are based on a chemical compound called 'benzodiazepines'. But even if emotional distress is not a phenomenon uniquely restricted to a modern way of life, its chemical solution is of a fairly recent date. Psychotropics constitute the term for a larger group of drugs which today are used by physicians to influence the central nervous system of the sufferer. Some drugs have a stimulating effect, others a tranquillising one. Related to their pharmacological effect and severity of symptoms, psychotropics are classified into four major groups: (1) antidepressants which are prescribed for depression; (2) neuroleptics which are prescribed for a range of psychotic symptoms, including schizophrenia; (3) tranquillisers which are prescribed for anxiety; and (4) hypnotics-sedatives which are used to ameliorate insomnia. The two former drug categories are prescribed for more severe psychiatric symptomatology, whereas the latter two – generally referred to as 'minor tranquillisers' – are prescribed for minor symptoms of anxiety and insomnia. Psychotropics are all prescribed drugs, which means that a person has to visit a physician and be given a prescription in order to have access to these drugs. A prolonged use requires that the user renews the prescription with a physician. Hence, when we in this book write about 'use' of psychotropics, we refer to legal drug use authorised by a physician. Only when specifically indicated do we discuss abuse, misuse or illegal use of psychotropics.

Although chemical coping with emotional states is nothing new, its introduction as a part of the therapy used by the medical profession is of rather recent date. Experimentations with clinical populations preceded by a few decades the final introduction of tranquillisers on to the commercial market in 1960 (Smith 1991). When psychotropics were made commercially available in the early 1960s, there was little concern about their negative aspects. They were instead considered as opening a new era in caring for people with both grave and minor mental health problems. The availability of psychotropic drugs gave further impetus to the reform movement in mental health care that had emphasised a gradual deinstitutionalisation of those suffering from mental illness. The adoption of drug therapy (like antipsychotic drugs) was thought to constitute a more humane treatment of patients cared for previously in mental institutions. The minor tranquillisers (i.e. drugs based on benzodiazepine derivatives like Valium and Librium) soon began to be widely used in the general population for treatment of anxiety and insomnia. Table 1.1 shows the main groups of the minor tranquillisers and their generic names, brand names and year of introduction. Over the past 20 years, the widespread use of psychotropics as quick mood modifiers and, specifically, the potential for abuse and dependency on benzodiazepines have become an area of concern for scholars in a variety of fields (Cappell et al. 1986; Gudex 1991). Although women tend to use these drugs twice as often as men, the gendered character of use has, thus far, not been raised as an issue of special interest. This book addresses the gender aspect of psychotropic drug use, problematises it and provides a theoretical framework for understanding it.

During the 1980s, social scientists addressed the social and cultural aspects of psychotropic drug use, thereby making the area a legitimate one of research and expertise within the social sciences. For example, in contrast to the previous

Table 1.1 Benzodiazepine derivatives: generic names, brand names, manufacturer and year of introduction

Generic name	Brand name	Manufacturer	Year of introduction
Chlordiazepoxide	Librium	Roche	1960
Diazepam	Valium	Roche	1963
Nitrazepam	Mogadon	Roche	1965
Oxazepam	Serenid-D	Wyeth	1966
Medazepam	Nobrium	Roche	1971
Lorazepam	Ativan	Wyeth	1972
Flurazepam	Dalmane	Roche	1974
Triazolam	Halcion	Upjohn	1979
Fluritrazepam	Rohypnol	Roche	1982
Alprazolam	Xanax	Upjohn	1983

mapping of the socio-demographic characteristics of users in the research of the 1970s (Cooperstock and Parnell 1982), there have been sociological accounts of the social and cultural meanings of psychotropic drug use (Cooperstock and Lennard 1979; Helman 1981; Gabe and Thorogood 1986; Montagne 1988, 1991), of pathways to use (Cafferata and Meyers 1990), and of how tranquillisers have become a public issue and constructed as a social problem in Britain (Gabe and Bury 1988, 1991a, 1991b; Gabe et al. 1991).

THE NEED FOR A GENDER-SENSITIVE PERSPECTIVE

This book is based on the assumption that, regardless of the value in offering a sociological perspective as an accompaniment to the medical perspective dominant in the field, a gender-sensitive perspective, more specifically a feminist perspective, has, however, been lacking among the new contributions provided by social scientists (eg. Gabe 1991a, 1991b). Although the sociological contributions in the field have challenged the notion of psychotropic drug use as a medically given matter, gender has not been problematised. We argue that, in order to understand psychotropic drug use, one has not only to problematise this use as a medical category but also the social category of gender. In our view, scholars must look at the intricacies of how illness is socially constructed as well as how sex and gender mix within oppressive social structures.

A problematisation of gender in the field of psychotropics has been hampered mainly for two reasons. First, the body, including its illnesses and sicknesses, were for a long time the sole prerogatives of the inquiries of the natural sciences, including medicine (Turner 1984). When sociologists began to examine health behaviour and sickness, they were even themselves unsure about the status of their enterprise. While the division between sociology *of* and *in* medicine for a while settled the dispute, the integration of the concerns of health seemed to have provided the sociologists with a domain of their own. Hence, as even the representatives of the mainstream of medical sociology were unsure of the status of their enterprise, it is not surprising that the voices of women's concerns were left unnoticed.

Second, research on illness and health behaviour, of which drug use is a part, has been heavily embedded in the functionalist perspective provided in Parsons' analysis of the sick role and the physician as the legitimiser of this role (Parsons 1951). (These ideas will be discussed in more detail in Chapters 3 and 4.) In Parsons' original account, both the physician and the patient were described in masculine terms, although he proposed a gender-neutral theory of human action. In Parsons' (1951:447) words, the physician's role 'centers on *his* responsibility for the welfare of the patient in the sense of facilitating *his* recovery from illness' (our emphasis). Later research has typically assigned the sick role to women as indeed empirical research tends to verify (Nathanson 1975; Verbrugge 1989). The paradox therefore is that, in the area of medical sociology, one can hardly accuse sociologists of not making women visible. In fact, the stereotypical female middle-aged patient with vague complaints is the typical 'problem' patient for the physician (Lorber 1975), while for researchers she has become an odd phenomenon since she lives longer than the men despite her ill health (Verbrugge 1985, 1989).

Interest in women's health issues in the 1980s has added new empirical knowledge to the gender-neutral research on ill health of the past (Roberts 1991a, 1991b; Verbrugge 1985, 1989). Furthermore, recent feminist contributions to the analysis of the social construction of women's health and illness (Martin 1989; Daly 1990; Riessman 1992) have highlighted the need to examine the social and cultural context of medicine and medical practice as well as the social construction of gender and illness. Yet, little of this research has found its way into the new social science perspective on psychotropic drug use. In short, gender-neutral research and naturalistic assumptions about the character of gender differences in health have hampered the production of a feminist knowledge of psychotropic drug use.

A gender-sensitive perspective not only makes gender visible but problematises existing gender relations and gender as a social institution (Stanley 1990:3–15; Harding 1991; Lorber 1994). This means specifically that powerful gender processes and structures influence culturally, politically and economically the meaning of 'female' and 'male'; the groupings of 'men' and 'women'; and divisions between a private and a public domain of social life are not taken for granted but problematised and placed at the forefront of the analysis. In order to develop a feminist analysis of women's use of psychotropic drugs, one has to uncover the absent presence of women in past research. Women form a hidden category in most studies on psychotropic drug users but the results are left untheorised and taken for granted. It is necessary to review critically previous work in the field and to make visible the 'invisible paradigm' of male-oriented work. We argue in this book that gender differentials in psychotropic drug use are concrete manifestations of the institution of gender in society.

The main aim of this chapter is to begin to familiarise the reader with our topic; to offer a brief introductory review of the existing research on psychotropic drug use; to highlight the gender blindness and biases in this research; and to introduce the reader to our empirical study of psychotropic drug users from which ideas for this book emerged. First, we will review the early work on gender differences in tranquilliser use and offer a clarification of how the 'one-dimensional' accounts are presented in the explanations and conclusions. We analyse this work from a gender-sensitive perspective and frame these accounts according to what their authors propose with special reference to gender. In a related discussion, we will show that the predominant focus has been epidemiological, drawing attention to individual rather than structural levels of concern.

DOUBLE RATE OF CONSUMPTION AND ONE-DIMENSIONAL EXPLANATIONS

Since the late 1960s, research on psychotropic drug use has shown consistently that women tend to use these drugs twice as often as men. A review of this literature indicates certain trends in the ways in which this finding is explained. In the following review we will examine the varied conclusions that these authors have made regarding this gender difference in psychotropic drug use. Parry's (1968) report from the first wave of surveys on the use of psychotropic drugs by American adults revealed that women were represented by more than half of the users and that those affiliated to the Jewish religion had above average rates of use. Noting that there appeared to be an inverse relationship between use and escape drinking, Parry suggests that both for women and Jewish people there is a strong taboo against heavy or escape drinking. He concludes: 'For neither group, however, are there similar well-structured and traditional objections to the use of psychotropics' (Parry 1968:805). This conclusion is made without empirically testing the attitudes of both groups towards the two substitute substances. Additionally, the use of the notions, taboo and traditional objections, suggests the existence of powerful cultural norms recognised by the author. Nevertheless, these powerful norms appear to influence drug-using behaviour as well as to allocate a moral imperative not to drink for certain social groups. Assumptions about what is acceptable behaviour for women target women as a distinct social group and, furthermore, as being more prone to psychotropic drug use than men. Yet, these assumptions are not questioned by Parry.

Jasper Woodcock's (1970) survey of long-term psychotropic drug users appearing on general practitioners' lists in England found that a high proportion (75 per cent) of these users were women. His conclusion is:

> it would appear that the reliance upon psychotropic compounds is related to neither the attitude of general practitioners nor to the character of the environment but to some factor both more personal to the patient and more all-pervading in the community. Whatever this factor may be, it affects women more powerfully than men, and the old more powerfully than the young.
>
> (Woodcock 1970:174)

The hidden factor is not explored further or linked in any way to the structural position of powerlessness which women and old people occupy in society.

A national study of psychotropic drug use in British general practice by Parish (1971:16) reveals that the sex ratio of use is 2.14:1 female to male. In his conclusions, he poses a question rather than offers an explanation of these results when he says, 'These results highlight some interesting problems which require further research: Why are twice as many women as men prescribed psychotropic drugs? There can be no conclusions to a report such as this but only questions' (Parish 1971:72). Yet, this article has in the later literature been referred to as providing an explanation of the gender differences in psychotropic drug use.

In a much quoted article, Ruth Cooperstock (1971) attempted to provide an explanatory model of the gender differences in psychotropic drug use and suggested that: 'Women are permitted greater freedom than men in expressing feelings. Because of this women are more likely to perceive or recognise their feelings and more specifically to recognise emotional problems in themselves' (Cooperstock 1971:241). For Cooperstock women feel freer to bring these problems to the attention of physicians who 'expect that a higher proportion of female than male patients will need mood modifiers' (1971:241). While the important issue of the 'feminisation' of psychotropic drug use is implicit here, the appeal to sex-role theory as a thorough explanation of the gender differences in the use of these drugs is not adequate. Representatives of sex-role theory see women's drug behaviour as a product of their sex-role socialisation. Hence, drug behaviour is viewed as part of the sex role, almost naturalised, but unrelated to the issue of structural inequality built into the gender system.

The findings from Linn and Davis' (1971) study of 100 women psychotropic drug users in Los Angeles indicated the importance of two relatively independent socio-cultural factors: religious affiliation and reference group interaction. A discussion of their results relies heavily on the work of Parry (1968). Therefore, Linn and Davis (1971:339), following in the tracks of Parry, simply conclude that there is 'no structured objection' to the use of psychotherapeutic drugs by women and Jewish people. Here we see, as in Parry's early work, subtle, normative undertones in this type of explanation.

In a large national study of American adults, Parry and his colleagues found that usage rates for psychotropic drugs was 'substantially higher amongst women than among men' (Parry et al. 1973:782). The authors suggest 'tentative explanations' for this difference and note: 'among women, a greater likelihood of visiting the physician, biological differences associated with the reproductive cycle, demands and allowances characterising female social roles, and less use of alternative substances for coping with emotional distress, e.g. alcohol' (Parry et al. 1973:782). In retrospect, that this explanation was defined as 'tentative' reveals a certain ambivalence on the part of the authors. Here, we see evidence of yet another appeal to sex-role theory as an 'adequate' explanation of the gender difference finding.

Balter, Levine and Manheimer (1974) conducted a cross-national study of nine Western European countries in 1972. This study revealed a similar pattern: women used psychotropic drugs twice as often as their male counterparts. The scholars conclude:

> We are particularly impressed by the uniformity of the findings for age and sex across countries and still wonder to what extent the differences in rate of drug use between the sexes is a socio-cultural phenomenon. The impact of the feminist movements now ongoing in many countries may provide a partial answer in the years to come.
>
> (Balter et al. 1974:774)

Again, as is the case with the sex-role proponents, women's drug use is perceived as a question of female culture and certain values that women hold. In addition to implicitly containing a blaming the victim ideology, the conclusion presents the women's movement as grounded on cultural values rather than structural inequalities, explicit in the existing gender system.

In the context of earlier studies, Lader (1978) mentions the rate of women's usage of psychotropics, specifically minor tranquillisers, as being twice as high as men's usage. His explanation for this rate is couched in monetary terms:

> In cost effective terms tranquillisers are cheap. It is cheaper to tranquillise distraught housewives living in isolation in tower blocks with nowhere for their children to go play than to demolish these blocks and to rebuild on a human scale or even to provide play groups. The drug industry, the government, the pharmacist, the tax payer and the doctor all have vested interests in 'medicalising' socially determined stress responses.
>
> (Lader 1978:164)

Within this limited framework, the reader is unable, here, to consider further how and why it is that more women than men are represented in this social process of medicalising stress.

In their now classic article, 'Some social meanings of tranquilizer use', Cooperstock and Lennard (1979) reveal findings from a Canadian interview study of 68 psychotropic drug users in which 76 per cent of users were female. Explaining women's use, these authors say:

> the majority recognized that their continuing use related to a variety of role strains. The most common strains and conflicts mentioned by female informants revolved around their traditional roles as wife, mother, houseworker, while males tended to discuss conflicts regarding their work or work performance.
>
> (Cooperstock and Lennard 1979:344)

This explanation is, in fact, an extension of Cooperstock's earlier work. However, in this article, the authors' invocation of sex-role theory, albeit inadequate, is reached through an appeal to the concept of 'role conflicts' for women.

THE TYPES OF ADVOCATE

In the majority of the work cited above, the categories women, women's role and the gender system are taken for granted and remain unproblematic. Neither notion, women or the gender system, is placed as the main focus of the above authors' conclusions, while their analyses are one-dimensional and individualistic. Let us examine each issue separately. First, one-dimensional analyses provide a myopic view of research material. As limited analyses, they either neutralise women and the workings of the gender system or assume that women exist primarily as passive or expressive rather than as active or instrumental social actors in relation to men – a theme to be detailed further in a related discussion in Chapter 3. We use the term one-dimensional as opposed to multi-dimensional. For us, multi-dimensional analyses problematise gender and are carried out by examining critically the subtle, structural dynamics of gender. Second, the individualistic focus of research on psychotropic drug use implies an emphasis on the individual user rather than structural factors related to high use in certain social groups. In this context, analyses of women's psychotropic drug use should take their departure in the gender system and the gendered processes that explain use both in the lay and professional culture.

The above review of the conclusions of previous research demonstrates the need for structural or multi-dimensional analyses, taking into account the complexities of the lives of women psychotropic drug users. Let us look at the above conclusions in more detail in an attempt to analyse this work with a 'feminist gaze' (Gamman and Marshment 1988). Here, we suggest that the above proponents making claims about the gender difference in psychotropic drug use fall into four types: the 'no objections' advocates, the 'cautious, no answers' advocates, the 'women's role' advocates and the 'political' advocates.

First, we are told by the *'no objections' advocates*, the 'early' Parry (1968) Linn and Davis (1971), that for women there is no well-structured and traditional opposition to the use of psychotropics. No reference in this work is made to the unintended, public consequences of use for female users as a social group. These unintended public consequences refer specifically to the varied objections many women have when they experience the debilitating, sometimes addicting effects that psychotropic drugs have on their lives as female gendered subjects. The main focus of the analyses and conclusions implies that the social category women is homogenised. There is little scope for problematising the notion, difference, among women as a social group, regardless of the fact that religion is mentioned as a discriminating variable.

There are also the *'cautious, no answers' advocates*: Woodcock (1970) and Parish (1971). On the one hand, Woodcock (1970) suggests that there could be some personal and more pervading factor in the community explaining women's high usage. But the author provides us with no further reference to what this factor could be. On the other hand, Parish (1971) merely suggests further research to answer the gender difference question, regardless of the fact that this gender difference and high use by women is consistently noted in his massive work. Operating from one-dimensional analyses taking the gender system as a given, neither author is therefore able to draw conclusions sensitive to women users. The reader is left somehow short-changed and, furthermore, unable to draw his or her own conclusions because of the limitations of the data.

There are also the *'women's role' advocates* suggesting that women's roles are similar to the attributes of the female role in general (Cooperstock 1971); the 'demands of female social roles' (Parry *et al.* 1973) or the more specific role strains related to the demands of women's role in the domestic domain (Cooperstock and Lennard 1979) and these explain their high rate of psychotropic drug use. While these authors highlight women in their own analyses and hint at gender sensitivity, they operate within a notion of assumed gender-specific attributes and roles which women have. Here again, these authors, like the 'no objections' advocates, homogenise women. They tend to naturalise women's roles. Hence, no theory of gender relations is offered beyond sex-role theory, taken as a given.

Women's drug use is assumed to be part of their sex role and hence 'normal' for them. In this way, their drug use is normalised and explained.

Lastly, there are the *'political'* advocates, Balter et al. (1974) and Lader (1978), who see the gender difference in the use of psychotropic drugs within a conventional, political framework rather than a gender-sensitive perspective. For example, Balter et al. (1974), looking to the future, suggest that the gender difference may be a cultural phenomenon, to be changed at least partially by the political activity of future feminists. Furthermore, Lader (1978) also politicises the issue by suggesting that women, particularly poor women, are bought off to keep medical costs down and private profits up. For these authors, it is more expedient to look for answers on a political terrain rather than to de-construct the issues with a gender-sensitive awareness. To begin to de-construct the issues with gender sensitivity reveals the lack of power that many women psychotropic drug users experience and indeed confront in managing their position in both the class and gender system. That structural inequality is inherent in the gender system is not a concern of these political advocates.

Overall, the claims of the above authors do not provide the reader with a sense of the complexities of psychotropic drug use for women. While all authors look at women's high usage of psychotropic drugs with interest, their overly descriptive accounts lack a structural dimension informed by a gender-sensitive analysis.

AN EPIDEMIOLOGICAL APPROACH AND THE LACK OF STRUCTURE

The lack of a structural dimension in the above research can be explained by the epidemiological approach prevailing in much of the research on psychotropic drug use (Tognoni et al. 1981; Williams and Bellantuono 1991), focusing drug-using behaviour on individual users. From a sociological perspective, this type of approach is a form of what Mills (1959) calls 'abstracted empiricism' inclined to psychologism as well as being systematically ahistorical and non-comparative. For Mills (1959:79), abstracted empiricists make little use of the 'basic idea of historical social structure'. Related to this type of argument, Young (1980) has critically assessed stress research and noted its empiricist tendencies whereby all social processes and structures are reduced to the attributes of individuals. Furthermore, Graham (1990) contends that within the sociology of health and illness a material / structural model is needed to explain differences in health behaviour, and that epidemiological research with a focus on the individual is limited because many people, specifically women, assess their health behaviour in less individualistic ways.

Furthermore, although useful in mapping out specific factors related to ill health, an epidemiological approach tends to provide an unsatisfactory basis for understanding women's health. In an epidemiological analysis, gender is merely one of the many background variables used in finding the correlations between social attributes, roles and ill health. The epidemiological approach in the field of psychotropic drug research tends, as Young (1980:144) contends, in the stress discourse to provide 'untheorised lists of social circumstances associated with stress inputs'. Along with this author, we argue that past descriptive research tends to legitimate existing social arrangements, effectively shadowing the need for theoretical approaches crucial for highlighting the gender issue. In turn, women's needs in the area remain hidden. As the reader will see, this contention is a basic theme of this book.

THE EMPIRICAL STUDIES IN CONTEXT

The empirical studies reported in this book were set out as an exploratory investigation of some of the above-mentioned, neglected dimensions in past research. As feminist scholars and women sociologists, we had a keen interest in developing a perspective on psychotropic drug use which would make the problems and needs of women psychotropic drug users more visible than they had been in past research. Of course, many of the theoretical ideas developed during the course of our work together have informed the discussions presented in this book.

In one empirical study, we examined comparative samples of men and women psychotropic users in a south-western metropolitan area in Finland. The focus and methodology of our study will be discussed in more detail in Chapter 6. We were aware already that previous research has not been able to explore fully gender differences because either the focus of these studies has been mainly on women users or gender had been mainly one of many social background variables. We saw that our research therefore filled a current gap in the field. Our guiding research question was: Do women use psychotropic drugs differently from men?

This question is of particular interest in terms of the levels of consumption of psychotropic drugs in a context other than an Anglo-Saxon one which constitutes the background of most previous research. Here, Finland is an interesting case. For example, while women are twice as likely as men to be users of psychotropics in other Western societies, including the other Nordic countries, this has not been the case in Finland where there appear to be few if any gender differences in the self-reported use of psychotropic drugs (Riska and Klaukka 1984; Riska *et al.* 1993). We began our research as an attempt to clarify some of the reasons for the Finnish findings.

As we develop our theoretical perspectives in this book, we will rely on some of the qualitative data collected in this study. The words of our users will illustrate how they view certain aspects of their lives and, more importantly, how they experience psychotropic drugs. Through their accounts we attempt to provide an insider's perspective (Conrad 1990). When relevant, we will also use empirical data to highlight key issues from this work.

The other empirical study consists of a content analysis of psychotropic drug advertising in the major medical journals in the Nordic countries. The purpose of this study was to illustrate how advertising provides a cultural representation of the user and to explore the gendered character of this representation. This study is examined in detail in Chapter 5.

THE STRUCTURE OF THIS BOOK

This book is informed by work within the fields of medical sociology, women's studies and, in specific contexts, addiction studies. As the reader will find, we argue that a gender-sensitive perspective and a feminist critique of existing work are needed.

Thus far, in our introduction, we have contended that previous research on psychotropic drug use is individualistic and one-dimensional. We have demonstrated how the individualistic focus of these accounts draws attention to individual rather than structural levels of concern and makes gender invisible. In Chapter 2, we elaborate on this discussion and show how the 'individualising-the-actor and neutralising-the-gender-factor approach' is one shared by those speaking from within both the medical and sociological discourses. In these discourses, an individualistic focus is emphasised; women's drug and health behaviour is naturalised and powerful gender processes operating within personal and social relationships, social institutions such as the medical profession, the media, the educational system, the state and throughout civil society remain invisible. The social construction of the gender system, of which tranquilliser use is a part, remains totally out of focus. The fact that women have been found consistently to use psychotropic drugs more often than men is not a problem. The picture we are left with is that tranquilliser use is an emergent social problem, albeit not a gendered problem.

In Chapter 3, we provide a review of the social scientific perspectives on psychotropic drug use with the intention of focusing on two approaches – the user- and the provider-oriented. We examine the imbalance between the development of both orientations as well as the theoretical implications of this imbalance.

Chapter 4 focuses on the layers in the social construction of psychotropic drug use. Here, we attempt to build a theoretical framework and highlight various layers of analyses that emerge when one looks at this complex social issue.

Looking at how moods are represented and indeed gendered, Chapter 5 presents findings from a study of advertisements for psychotropics in major medical journals in the Nordic countries.

Chapters 6, 7 and 8 reveal findings which have emerged from one of our empirical studies, and the focus, in all three chapters, is on users as speaking subjects. Specifically, Chapter

6 explores the individual layer of analysis in the social construction of psychotropic drug use. In this exploration, the
concepts of the discursive subject and the narrative are used to
bring forth the sufferer's experience of ill health. Chapter 7
examines the group layer of analysis and explores uncomfortable moods within the context of the lay culture. Chapter 8
examines sufferers' links with the health care system. We aim
to provide a picture of the lay culture surrounding the use of
psychotropic drugs. With special reference to the field of
addiction studies, the concept of drug career is utilised as well
as amended. This concluding chapter introduces the concept
of dependency as a gendered issue and provides the final
touches to a comprehensive framework on psychotropic
drugs.

Throughout the discussions in this book, we attempt to
show that in the field of psychotropic drugs, a gender-
sensitive approach challenges the theoretical and methodological pitfalls explicit in previous research. We contend that
this type of approach problematises both men's and women's
use of these drugs. By pointing to both the complex structural
and cultured processes that are related to psychotropic drug
use, gender becomes visible. The structural aspects are addressed by signalling the importance of the interplay between
the private and the public domains of gender relations, the
dynamics of the gender system and its effects upon women.
The cultural aspects are addressed by problematising illness
and gender as socially constructed categories and society as a
system of gendered relationships, in which women more than
men are subverted by oppressive social practices.

That gender-insensitive studies on women psychotropic
drug users have been produced mainly by gender-blind
malestream thinkers reveals that the way in which problems
are conceptualised and what is studied are inextricably linked.
We wrote this book because we recognised the need to challenge malestream ways of thinking and to offer an alternative
approach in this area.

Chapter 2

New challenges

The medical and sociological discourses

INTRODUCTION

In this chapter, we outline with special reference to women the two predominant discourses on psychotropic drug use: the medical and the sociological. We offer a critical review of these two discourses visible in the field as well as argue that the current sociological discourse is gender blind and thus incapable of explaining the use of the predominant users, women – a theme which will be expanded in Chapter 3.

Here, we suggest that studies on psychotropics can be categorised into those which are gender sensitive and those which are gender blind. As implied earlier in Chapter 1, we define a gender-sensitive perspective on psychotropic drug use as one in which the categories of women and the gender system are not taken as given but problematised and placed at the forefront of the analysis. Furthermore, we contend that only when this distinction is made, will a broader understanding of women's use of drugs, specifically minor tranquillisers, be achieved. If a truly new understanding promised by social scientists in the past is to develop, paradigms prevailing in current research need to be questioned, dissected and complemented with an analysis that problematises the workings of gender.

THE MEDICAL AND SOCIOLOGICAL DISCOURSES

Traditional assumptions emerging chiefly from the medical

community, such as 'minor tranquillisers are safe and effective symptomatic remedies', 'the doctor–patient relationship is sacrosanct or above criticism' or 'the pharmaceutical industry is blameless or a benign facilitator for the organised health care system' (an assumption to be examined closely in Chapter 5), have been challenged as being 'false' or 'outdated' both by medical experts and by social scientists. These challenges have been presented by representatives of what we here will characterise as a medical discourse and a sociological discourse. By discourse, we mean simply a way of conceptualising the problem.

The medical discourse, based primarily on the claims of concerned representatives of the medical profession and pharmacologists, 'individualises' the issue of psychotropic drugs by drawing attention either to the utilisation, effects and consequences of these drugs for the recipients or to the extent and pattern of use within a specific health care delivery system, a particular society or across cultures. The representatives of the medical discourse interpret the rate of use as a public health concern and as evidence of a need for change in health care delivery. Thus, the conclusions drawn from this discourse become recommendations for the need for some level of change. But change here means technological modifications or procedural adjustments directed towards the level of health care provision rather than addressing the structural aspects of use.

The sociological discourse has been established by the claims of sociologists and anthropologists and informed by a societal perspective on psychotropic drug use. It employs notions such as 'social control'; 'social context and meaning of use'; 'public health consequences'; 'the management of everyday life'; 'medicalisation of stress'; 'the mobilisation of public opinion'; and 'the emergence of a social problem'. While these social dimensions of psychotropic drug use have the potential to become building blocks for a critical perspective, these dimensions have, so far, remained incapable of explaining women's use. This is because these authors extol 'subjective meaning', 'contextual theorising' or 'micro levels of concern' to the exclusion of 'structural dynamics', 'gender-sensitive theorising' and 'macro-levels of concern'. In the final analysis, the issues of power and structural transformation become irrelevant.

Overall, these discourses have existed in partnership rather than in opposition to each other. The sociological discourse has had a unique role to play in outlining the social problem of tranquilliser use as being distinct from the social consequences of that self-same use. In a powerful way, separating 'use' from 'consequences' makes a subtle, but clear analytical distinction between the 'private' and the 'public', a distinction necessary for the development of a feminist analysis. On the other hand, this distinction has consistently been constructed (as we shall see) on male-focused terrains. The social scientific constructions signify how use, although problematic, can be not only beneficial to the promotion of a public health model (a major concern of representatives of the medical discourse) but also 'theoretically' valuable in developing 'a social problem perspective' for the sociology of health and illness (a major concern of representatives of the sociological discourse).

In effect, the sociological and the medical discourses have a common approach with an underlying concern for recognising the public health and social consequences of psychotropic drug use. At first glance, this common approach may appear to be focused on a macro-level of concern or to include a structural dimension. However, drug-using behaviour remains on an individual level and there is a lack of understanding of the social processes and structures which produce differences in health behaviour. Given that the focus is on the individual, this approach is not only limited but also makes women invisible.

This, what we term 'individualising-the-actor and neutralising-the-gender-factor approach', provides an unsatisfactory basis for understanding women's use of psychotropic drugs. In order to develop a feminist account of psychotropic drug use, we will illustrate how the 'individualising-the-actor and neutralising-the-gender-factor approach' utilised within both the medical and sociological discourses has systematically excluded women. Here we argue that in psychotropic drug research an understanding of the importance of gender and the gender system and the various layers of help-seeking behaviour has been lacking. We examine first the medical discourse and then the sociological discourse on psychotropic drug use with their various strands of thinking. We contend that the development of a common approach rests on the foundation of malestream analyses. The resultant effect has been the barring of a gender-sensitive analysis in this subject area.

THE MEDICAL DISCOURSE ON PSYCHOTROPIC DRUG USE

Over the years, psychotropic drugs, particularly benzo-diazepines, have been identified as creating withdrawal symptoms and pharmacological and psychological dependence (Owen and Tyrer 1983; Petursson and Lader 1981; Cappell et al. 1986; Montagne 1991; Smith 1991; Gudex 1991; Medawar 1992). They have also been found to be frequently abused by chemically dependent patients (DuPont 1990). While there is a wide range of these drugs available, it has been suggested that the need for benzodiazepines could be met by one or two compounds (Summers et al. 1990; Medawar 1992).

The medical discourse has been focused primarily on the individual benefits of psychotropic drug use for the patient and the doctor's need for what Lader (1991:93) has referred to as 'thoughtful prescribing'. There is little hint that the medical discourse upholds the use of these drugs as 'medicalising everyday life' (Mondanaro 1989) or as a 'means of social control' (Koumjian 1981). Indeed, these drugs are viewed as necessary and an essential part of the medical armamentarium of drugs. In essence, the main theme of this discourse is that these drugs are valuable to the individual patient, a sufferer from anxiety and insomnia, needing this type of pharmacological support. The problem is *not* the medication but its improper use. With this emphasis, the medical discourse has been unable to explain the complex reasons why women more than men are involved in a type of health behaviour that has the potential to damage rather than promote their health. Additionally, there is no analysis offered as to why women more than men pursue lifestyles needing pharmacological supports.

For example, although a high level of psychological

dependency was found among 'present long-term users' in Murray's (1981:857) study, drug taking was seen by these users 'as a means of sustaining life rather than a determinant course of treatment'. In later work, Murray and her colleagues (Murray *et al.* 1982:1597) found 'high prevalence of both physical and psychological ill health in the sample . . . and little evidence of heavy reliance on either the doctor or medicines'. The former finding had also been noted by Clare (1981) in a previous context. Here, patients' needs, whether physical or psychological, were upheld as the determining factor of use.

Around that time, Marks (1982), a consistent opponent of the medicalisation view, accused sociologists of shifting this 'patient' emphasis to the effects of these drugs rather than the patient's need for them. He claims that 'the social implication of drug therapy is still in its infancy and the literature tends to be sprinkled with *ex cathedra* comments from sociologists, predominantly expressing fears about drug effects' (Marks 1982:351). In a later context he says, 'there is no evidence that such use reduces the appropriate reaction to the social ills that cause the stress, nor that drugs are being given for social problems' (p. 352). His solution is that the presenting problems can best be reduced by 'appropriate education of doctors' (p. 350) and, implicitly, sociologists.

A year later, in a less authoritative tone, Marks (1983:142) says that 'Before deciding that the prescribing practices of physicians are reasonable so far as benzodiazepines are concerned, it is important to make sure that their use is not reducing the search for social solutions to these stress disorders.' Marks' later emphasis is a hidden warning to overprescribing physicians and an indication that the simultaneous claims of sociologists (as we will soon see) are being heard.

On the other hand, a lone voice in this discourse comes from Hansen (1989), a pharmacologist who sees the use of benzodiazepines for social and everyday problems as being perplexing. For her, benzodiazepine use is 'another side of the chemical curtain's effect which locks the user in a problematic situation and makes benzodiazepine usage a form of social control' (Hansen 1989:166). As a female pharmacologist,

Hansen is a part of the medical discourse. Nevertheless, she makes an opposing claim as her writing is sensitive to gender.

More recently, a defence of the medical discourse has been offered by Lader (1991:93) who contends that 'primary care practitioners are becoming increasingly adept at exploiting techniques to cope with anxiety disorders without resorting to tranquillisers.' Given that Lader does not outline what these medical techniques are, it is difficult to assess whether or not these techniques are valuable from the consumer's point of view.

As we have seen from the discussion above, the medical discourse has focused primarily on the relative benefits of psychotropic drug use. Specifically, 'benzodiazepines have become regarded by medical practitioners and patients alike as safe and effective remedies' (Lader 1991:90). At most, research in this area points to the limitations of clinical medicine. However, it appears that these limitations can be overcome by vigilance and attentiveness on the part of pre-scribing physicians. It is assumed that the physicians rather than the patients have the power to overcome these existing drawbacks. There is no question that individual sufferers of anxiety and insomnia may not need this type of pharma-cological aid. Although some studies consider what may be helpful psychologically in order to withdraw from psycho-tropics (e.g. sympathetic listening, anxiety management and behaviour therapy), these interventions are viewed as being outside of the medical discourse which is unable to offer an integrated approach (Hamlin and Hammersley 1989a, 1989b). Furthermore, the fact that the majority of the sufferers are women is not seen as a problem. In this regard, the medical discourse offers individualistic and gender-insensitive explan-ations of use.

THE SOCIOLOGICAL DISCOURSE ON PSYCHOTROPIC DRUG USE

A concern for social consequences of use

Alongside the medical discourse has existed a sociological discourse which has interpreted the issue of dependence on psychotropic drugs as part of the 'widespread questioning of the role of medical treatments' (Gabe and Bury 1991b:453). The argument here is that criticism of the use of these drugs is part of a general crisis in medicine, a crisis in which doubts about developments within medical practice are reflected. The representatives of the sociological discourse have illuminated some of the social and cultural processes which problematise dependence on drugs and more specifically define psychotropic drug use as a distinct social problem. Within this discourse, drug intervention is viewed as a quick cure for many social ills (Gottlieb 1975) and the widespread use of benzodiazepines as an extension of the idea of a 'culture of technology' (Porpora 1986).

Moreover, the sociological discourse has provided information about the linkage of psychotropic drugs to a variety of individual, interpersonal and social levels: to an individual user's need for chemical comforts (Helman 1981; Gossop 1988); doctors' love affairs with tranquillisers (Mondanaro 1989); tranquillisers as a form of social control (Koumjian 1981); the tranquillising of society (Sterling 1989); and the penetration of these drugs on the illicit market with the resultant abuse by injecting drug users (Black 1988). More recently, detailed information on the relationship between gender and pathways to psychotropic drug use has been provided (Cafferata and Meyers 1990).

In this context, Cooperstock and Parnell published in 1982 a comprehensive review of research on psychotropic drug use. In their evaluation of this research, they conclude: 'The benzodiazepines may be viewed like alcohol as social drugs. From an epidemiological perspective, this new definition demands a re-conceptualization of the consequences of use of these drugs, and hence a more diversified approach to research' (Cooperstock and Parnell 1982:1192). Here, while recognising the importance of epidemiology and, implicitly, the medical discourse, these authors attempt to focus the debate on an intellectual 'meeting ground' for the medical and social discourses. 'Public health consequences' become their overriding concern. They continue: 'Given this broad conceptual framework, both the negative physical and social effects of these drugs would be viewed as public health issues' (Cooperstock and Parnell 1982:1192).

Additionally, by focusing on tranquilliser use as social control and ultimately the tranquilliser issue as a social problem, representatives of the sociological discourse reflect a shared concern with their counterparts in the medical discourse. This concern is to consider the social consequences of use as being equal to the public health consequences of psychotropic drug use. But this underlying concern is based on a gender blindness evident in both the medical and the sociological discourses. Continuing our examination of the sociological discourse, we will next look at a shift from an emphasis on tranquillisers as social control to an emphasis on tranquillisers as a social problem and, ultimately, the implications of this shift for women.

Tranquillisers as social control

Waldron (1977) presents a strong case for the medicalisation or social control view in one of the first important discussions in the sociological discourse. She suggests that prescribing drugs to a patient, who is distressed by psychological and social problems, is in many cases not medically justified; that the use of benzodiazepines can be identified with a trend in society which tends to medicalise the problems of everyday life; and that prescriptions for these drugs increased rapidly during the 1960s and 1970s, a period of increasing social problems. Waldron (1977:43) speculates further that the 'medicalization of these [social and economic problems] reduces pressures for societal change and this outcome is advantageous from the point of view of those who profit from the existing economic and political order.' Implicitly, Waldron attempts, by focusing on the macro-level, to 'raise' the issue of prescribed drug use to the level of a social problem alongside alcoholism, suicide and homicide. Waldron's arguments lack, however, a clear theoretical foundation. This is primarily because the majority of her arguments are based on an unstated assumption: there is a 'hidden alliance' between the medical profession, the pharmaceutical industry and the state.

In a similar vein of thought, Koumjian (1981) sees the use of Valium, a minor tranquilliser, as a means of social control and involved in the medicalisation of everyday life. Koumjian observes that these drugs are frequently prescribed to old people, women and those in lower socio-economic groups. Koumjian's analysis is a convincing account because his identifiable, most frequently prescribed groups can be viewed as traditionally powerless groups in society – the elderly, women and the poor. Koumjian does suggest that the purpose of control emerges from social concerns. However, his arguments lack a theory of social agency, in which the social actions of individuals are problematised and thus included within a structural or macro-level analysis.

As the sociological discourse on social control develops, the claims being made about 'control' become linked with individual rather than structural concerns. Simply, whether the emphasis is on social consequences (i.e. in terms of social control or social problems) or, more subtly, on social meaning, the research practice of social scientists has been to focus on the individual level as the main analytical site. This focus on micro-level concerns is a shared form of conceptualising in the medical and sociological discourses. At the same time, structural issues such as power, gender, race and class and the interplay between these issues are increasingly neglected in sociological analyses, focusing on tranquillisers as social control.

For example, aware that within the social control view 'blame has been laid at many doors', Helman (1981:521) chooses to focus on the individual user. In a fascinating account, he looks at the social and symbolic meaning of long-term psychotropic drug use and, perhaps more importantly, he attempts to explain the 'perceived' control of the patient over his or her drugs by the use of metaphors. This work evidences a shift in emphasis from 'control of the patient by the doctor' to 'control over the drug by the patient'. Regardless of whether the symbolic use of tranquillisers is, for the patient, a tonic, fuel or food, the key discriminating factor is how the patient exhibits control over the use of the drug. For Helman, this spectrum of control ranges from self-medication (tonic), to variable control for social conformity (fuel) and finally to little control (food). While social control is not an explicit theme in this work, Helman's findings are provocative given that the 'food' group, exhibiting the least control of their drugs and being most dependent upon doctors, unlike the other groups, is 100 per cent female. But an explanation of the latter finding cannot be found in Helman's work.

Clearly, Helman's work illustrates specifically gender blindness. On the one hand, gender has an absent presence, emerging from the data: women are consistently and predominantly the research subjects. On the other hand, data on the gender factor are subsumed or made invisible by data on 'symbolic meaning', viewed by Helman as the most important factor. Most importantly, that women's use of psychotropic drugs and the issue of 'food' are linked in Helman's work is indeed significant. By this time, gender-sensitive work (Orbach 1978) had already identified women's relationship to food as problematic. Hence, Helman's lack of a discussion on the implications of the link between psychotropic drug use and its symbolic meaning as food for women disregards the gender issue.

Along with these authors, Gabe and Lipshitz-Phillips (1984:538), challenging the view that tranquillisers are a form of social control, contend that this view is 'too mechanistic' and has resulted in 'over-generalisations'. Within the framework of their empirical case study, they then proceed to demonstrate quite convincingly that there is little support for the ways in which benzodiazepines are involved in the medicalisation of everyday life. In analysing benzodiazepine prescribing and its use as a possible form of social control, they consider five issues: doctors' power, patient dependence, gender and class ideology, the oversocialised view of the person, and the limits of functionalism.

By constant reference to their own data, they systematically attempt to demolish earlier claims that tranquillisers are a form of social control. In effect, they call for 'theoretical modifications' and 'a model which treats social control as context dependent and not something to be assumed in advance' (Gabe and Lipshitz-Phillips 1984:542). Nevertheless, it is important to point out two fundamental problems in this work – the first methodological and the second theoretical.

First, while these authors state that 'the data on gender and class can be used to support or reject the social control thesis' (Gabe and Lipshitz-Phillips 1984:537), they opt for the latter course of action in their final construction of the data without giving sufficient explanation. Their justification for this course of action is that there are 'several ways of interpreting' the data on social class and gender and they offer what they call 'counter interpretations'. This is problematic. When both interpretations and counter interpretations from the data are brought out as simultaneously supporting the authors' main conclusion (that tranquillisers are not a form of social control), the conclusions themselves become equivocal. While the authors justify this methodological strategy by claiming the need to be 'contextual', the only conclusion that can be drawn is that within the conclusion is a 'counter conclusion' which itself is contextual (that tranquillisers are a form of social control).

Second, it must be remembered that, while the authors consider how their data contradict the social control argument with regard to a series of five theoretical issues, the issues that the authors select and in turn discuss are self-chosen and not necessarily empirically based. It could be argued that two of the most important issues implicit in the social control debate have been gender and class. Nevertheless, in their discussion, the authors relegate these issues to a single theoretical category, 'gender and class ideology', and thus prioritise micro-level (individual) rather than macro-level (structural) concerns. Furthermore, the theoretical absence of the notions of gender, class and indeed race in their discussions about doctors' power, patients' dependence, the oversocialised view of the person and the limits of functionalism is perhaps a glaring omission.

Still, Gabe's further work (Gabe and Thorogood 1986), inclusive of the issue of race, does succeed on the sociological terrain in re-conceptualising some of the consequences of use of these drugs for white women and women of colour. In our view, this later work does open the way for a more diversified sociological approach to research. For example, the authors recognise the importance of contextual theorising; the social context of tranquilliser use alongside the management of everyday life; and the use of these drugs as a resource. Nevertheless, they explicitly reject the social control viewpoint. It is obvious that their main analytical site is gendered (i.e. they are studying women), but their subjects, women, remain limited within individual or micro-level concerns. A concern for gender and its social organisation is in a sense sacrificed for a concern for the factors of class and race. Thus, many questions concerning the 'feminisation' of illness and, in turn, tranquilliser use as a gendered attribute remain unanswered.

Tranquilliser use as a social problem

Ultimately, the above work has laid the groundwork for a strand of thinking in the 'social problems arena', while at the same time conceptualising the 'consequences of use' as a public health issue.

When Gabe and Bury (1988) asserted that the excessive use of legally prescribed drugs represents a form of social behaviour that falls on the margins between deviance and normality, they attempted to demolish further the social control debate and to transform key issues to a more neutral territory: a debate focused on social problems. Indeed, to conceptualise the misuse of prescribed drugs from a social problem stand-point has the dual advantage of developing a certain level of theoretical (sociological) sophistication, while sharing a concern and approach with members of the medical discourse. This shared concern based on social problems 'in the context of public health' is not contested. A focus on the social context of use is valued, while attention is fixed on the somewhat un-foreseen consequences of the mobilisation of public opinion by the media and the state's response (Bury and Gabe 1990, 1991). Hence, the once heated debate about social control between members of the medical and the sociological discourses has abated. A consensus is achieved: tranquilliser use is identified as an emergent social problem but not a gendered problem. Most importantly, the social problem is tacitly the female psychotropic drug user. We contend that women tranquilliser users receive little benefits, if any, from being labelled a social problem, with deviant implications. (This issue will be discussed in more detail in Chapter 8.)

In the final analysis, women tranquilliser users with their attributed status as a social problem become, now more than ever before, open to public surveillance. This type of analysis creates the equation, 'Drug use as a social problem equals women'. Transgressing women and not the gender system are the focus of attention. Given that tranquilliser use is conceptualised as an emergent, gender-neutral social problem, the need for the gender dimension of this issue to be made visible and problematised becomes urgent.

In the above discussion on the sociological discourse on psychotropic drug use, we saw how this particular discourse has developed various strands of thinking, from one focusing on tranquilliser use as social control to one identifying the tranquilliser issue as a social problem. In other words, the notion 'social problem', along with its specific theoretical framework and conceptual baggage, gradually begins to take priority over the notion 'social control'. Simply, social problem rather social control becomes imperceptibly established as a primary signifier of the use of tranquillisers in society. Tranquilliser use, a newly found social problem, emerges as gender neutral, regardless of the fact that women more than men continue to consume these drugs. These discussions demonstrate clearly that a gender-sensitive perspective is absent among the recent contributions provided by sociologists in the field.

CONCLUSION

We have contended that previous research on psychotropic drug use is gender biased, gender blind and one-dimensional. We have demonstrated how the individualistic focus of these accounts, whether medical or sociological, draws attention to individual rather than structural levels of concern and makes gender invisible. We contended that an 'individualising-the-actor and neutralising-the-gender-factor approach' is one shared by those speaking from within both the medical and sociological discourses. The fact that women have been found consistently to use psychotropic drugs more than men is not perceived as problematic. We are only left with the idea that tranquilliser use is an emergent social problem, without reference to the structural inequalities which produce that problem for women. The construction of the gender system, of which tranquilliser use is a part, remains totally out of focus.

In the next chapter we build on this framework and focus specifically on the main theoretical orientations within a sociological perspective.

Chapter 3

Social scientific perspectives
The 'users' and the 'providers'

INTRODUCTION

The purpose of this chapter is to provide an overview of the approaches in the social scientific research on psychotropic drug use. As will be demonstrated in this chapter, these approaches can be analysed in terms of the major actor involved – depicted as the major initiator of drug consumption – and of the theoretical framework used to interpret the results on drug use. While the former approach can be described as user- or provider-oriented studies, a majority of these studies tends to focus on *the user*. In this respective work, the term, user, denotes a generic concept for the aggregation of individuals, who on the basis of self-reported use in surveys have been found to share a common attribute, such as gender, age, income, ill health.

The other 'actor' focus prevalent in studies on psychotropic drug use is on the *provider*, either the prescribing physician or the pharmaceutical industry. One version holds that physicians are merely social control agents and drug prescribing is part of controlling individuals. Still another version of this perspective holds that the driving motive behind the pharmaceutical industry is increased profits in the sales of psychotropic drugs, and the prescribing physician is simply a puppet in the profit-making efforts of the international pharmaceutical giants. It is only more recently that the mediating cognitive structures between the user and the provider have been explored. In attempts to understand the workings of such cognitive structures, sociologists have pointed to the prevailing medical discourse and the role of drug advertising as a form of cultural representation. In the following two sections, we will provide an account of the sociological approaches which have focused on the user or the provider. In this review, we will present the theoretical frameworks which have been used to explain research results. We argue that the theoretical perspectives tend to be invisible and, generally, can be identified only through authors' basic assumptions and concepts inherent in their research design or in descriptions of their findings.

USER-ORIENTED PERSPECTIVES

As Chapters 1 and 2 show, a growing body of research in various Western countries has provided information about the social profile of users over the past two decades. The initial research included valuable information about the prevalence of psychotropic drug use in various population groups. The studies show remarkably similar results regardless of country: for example, use increases with age and is more common among women than men. Much of this research has been descriptive and repeatedly the sociological framework provided has been salient. In those user-oriented studies where a theoretical framework can be discerned, three theoretical perspectives can be identified. First, the functionalist perspective dominates a large part of the early research done on psychotropic drug use. Within this framework, psychotropic drug use is seen as part of illness behaviour and the sick role. Second, a perspective focusing on structural factors gained ground in the late 1970s and 1980s. Third, and more recently, a social constructionist account has become visible in studies on psychotropic drug use.

The functionalist perspective on psychotropic drug use

The functionalist perspective has a long tradition in sociology and was the dominant framework in medical sociology until the early 1970s, when Marxist and social constructionist approaches began to gain ground. The early sociological accounts of illness behaviour in the field of medical sociology were inspired by Parsons' (1951) classic work on the sick role and the role of the physician in legitimating the sick role.

The basic assumption underlying the Parsonian sick-role concept is that illness and health are not merely biological categories, but parts of a social system. Individuals are expected to fulfil their social roles and meet the normative requirements as well as expectations related to their social roles. The sick role is an institutionalised solution offered to the individual when, because of involuntary reasons, such as illness, he or she cannot perform his or her role properly. Hence, the sick role is a social mechanism whereby a deficient role performance, not having a basis in the individual's free will, is regulated in society. The medical profession acts as a regulator of this kind of involuntary, temporary 'deviancy'. Its task is to ensure that the patient is returned to an optimal level of role performance.

A social system approach, including the above views on the sick role and the medical profession, characterised much of Parsons' work after the 1950s (Swingewood 1993; Gerhardt 1989). Here, the focus is on social systems and the mechanisms of social integration. Pattern variables become the central concepts whereby Parsons describes the value orientations that govern an individual's – in our case the doctor's and the patient's – behaviour. Clusters of common norms and values are internalised and provide a shared framework for human actions.

Parsons' structure of action was, however, guided by different value orientations, prevailing in various spheres or systems. Pattern variables explain the values guiding the role of a professional in modern society, while the physician's behaviour was portrayed as the prototype of professional behaviour. Gender roles were part of the private sphere and the family – roles which became synonymous with sex roles in the early sociology of the family. Sex-role theory presents the female role as 'expressive' and caring for the home, while the male role is 'instrumental' and oriented towards work outside the family unit. In Parsons' (1942) own account, these expected roles are more conflict-laden than the harmonious picture provided in later sociological literature. Furthermore, a serious reading of Parsons does not render unequivocal support for the later growth of sex-role theory. Further developments of this theory are, in our view, based on a simplistic notion of sex roles, concerning women's behaviour and, in this context, will be called the *'women-are-expressive' hypothesis.*

The gender differences in illness behaviour – women being ill more often and using health services more frequently – were in early mainstream, medical sociology attributed to men's and women's sex-role behaviour. This interpretation of gender differences in ill health has also been referred to as the 'compatibility hypothesis' (Gerhardt 1989:280). According to this hypothesis, the female sex role is compatible with the adoption of a sick role (Cooperstock 1971; Nathanson 1975). Here, it is assumed that women are more inclined than men to adopt the sick role because women are allowed by society to show their emotions and, additionally, are more willing than men to acknowledge their symptoms. Not only are women thought to have a lower threshold for seeing a physician, but also it is assumed that women have 'more time' to engage in the sick role than men (Nathanson 1975, 1977).

In effect, women's higher rate of psychotropic drug use in comparison to men's has mainly been attributed to prevailing sex roles. The gender characteristics of women – their assumed expressiveness – have been presented as the reason for women's inclination to perceive and express emotional problems to which the physician responds by prescribing psychotropics (Cooperstock 1971; Cafferata *et al.* 1983:132–3). Much of the early survey research on users of psychotropics took the 'women-are-expressive' hypothesis for granted. This hypothesis became *in itself* an explanation for gender differences in use rather than an hypothesis to be tested.

Applying sex-role theory to explain gender differences in psychotropic drug use has resulted in a number of conceptual problems. First, and most strikingly, although sex-role theory provides an adequate description of gender differences in psychotropic drug use, it takes gender roles as given categories, including the specific attitudes and problems attached to these categories. No explicit distinction is made between the category of sex and gender in discussions of these categories. As a result, differences between them tend to be blurred. Some analysts see gender construction as the link between culture and nature. In this context, we adhere to Butler's (1993:5) notion that 'nature' also has a history and that 'the social construction of the natural presupposes the cancellation of the natural from the social'. In Butler's (1993:2) own words gender is a 'cultural construct' and sex is 'a norm which qualifies a body for life within the natural intelligibility'.

A second and related problem is that, within sex-role theory, the female attribute of expressiveness is taken for granted in women as a sex category. Similarly, women's ill health is presented as a 'normal' and, thus, 'natural' condition for them. By normalising and naturalising women's ill health, social scientists have trivialised its expression and etiology. In the same way, a high prevalence of psychotropic drug use has been 'normalised' for women: they are expressive and more prone to shifting moods. Hence, it is normal for women to need mood modifiers. There are two notions included within this conceptualisation, which will be shown to appear frequently in the literature on psychotropic drug use. The first notion is the naturalistic belief in a presocial, biological basis of gender roles. Sex-role theory provides no explanation of why stereotypical sex roles exist and continue to be maintained other than their functionality and basis in a normative consensus. Ultimately, this explanation falls back to a reductionistic view: sex roles are reduced to biological differences rather than being socially constructed categories of gender and an intricate part of the institutionalised gender system.

The second notion is that there are gender-based adaptation mechanisms to anxiety and stress. It is assumed that women resort to the legal drug-using culture as part of a feminine subculture in modern society. Although distinct cultural processes are pregnant in this explanation, the analysis is generally presented in terms of the 'normality' of women's illness behaviour. Therefore, this behaviour is naturalised – located in the sphere of the presocial rather than in society.

A third shortcoming of the sex-role theory as an explanation of gender differences in psychotropic drug use is the perpetuation of stereotypical notions of women's and men's behaviour. The notion that women have 'more time' than men to engage in the sick role implies that women's work in the home is viewed as a form of leisure activity – merely emotional work rather than, or including, arduous physical labour. To view women's work in the domestic domain as mainly emotional work, a 'labour of love', conceals both the physical work involved in the caring function as well as women's economic dependency on men (Graham 1983, 1984). Some scholars (e.g. Waldron 1977; Suffet and Brotman 1976; Christie 1984) have explicitly suggested that the subordinated and dependent position of the traditional housewife or women in general is the major reason for women's use of psychotropics. The merits of this viewpoint are that it problematises women's use, while identifying the gender system as a key structural condition related to women's psychotropic drug use.

While the 'women-are-expressive' hypothesis has been used as an interpretative framework for women's high rate of psychotropic drug use, men's lower level of use has been explained by another, gender-specific hypothesis – the *substitution hypothesis*. The latter hypothesis proposes that men use psychotropic drugs less often than women because men self-medicate most common, everyday stresses and anxieties by using alcohol (e.g. Parry *et al.* 1974). This hypothesis is based on a functionalist interpretation which assumes that all human beings have a need for a relaxation-producing psychoactive substance (see, for example, Bell 1980; Kalant 1980:11). This universal need is seen to be channelled into different routes for both men and women in modern society. Gender-specific norms in society have created gender-specific functional alternatives. Men have traditionally used alcohol as a relaxation-producing substance but, during the past century, this substance use has been viewed in negative terms for women. As social historians have pointed out, women were themselves active in constructing these norms in an effort to control men's alcohol use during the era of the temperance movement and Prohibition (Gusfield 1963; Levine 1980).

When psychotropics emerged on the commercial market in the 1960s, there were no explicit cultural norms prohibiting women from using these psychoactive substances. On the contrary, tranquillisers confirmed the traditional passive and subordinate female role (Christie 1984). Women, trying to break sex-role expectations, did not have to be declared mentally ill and confined to mental institutions, as in the past. They had the possibility of being kept docile, tamed or obedient with the assistance of psychotropic drugs (Fisher 1986:153). It should be noted that this latter, feminist viewpoint is contrary to the consensual view of gender relations offered within the traditional functionalist perspective.

The substitution hypothesis suggests, therefore, that psychotropics and alcohol are two gender-specific, socially legitimate substances that have equivalent functions. This notion of equivalent chemical coping mechanisms conceals, however, the basic contextual differences between men's and women's use of substances. Men can themselves initiate their use of alcohol, while there is a social context (i.e. the pub, a party, etc.) as well as a shared cultural code regulating their alcohol consumption. Women, by contrast, cannot themselves initiate their use of psychotropics, if they are not receiving these substances from professionals. In the case of legal psychotropic use, the doctor prescribes and determines the dosage and duration of the regimen. Furthermore, women, in contrast to men, lack a shared social context and cultural code that would provide a collective definition and regulation of their drug consumption. Since their use of psychotropics tends to take place in private, such norms are unlikely to emerge. Similarly, while men have a shared vocabulary of experiencing and describing the intoxicating effects of alcohol, women have no common language to express their dependency on psychotropics. Recent public debates on the dependency-producing effects of benzodiazepines have resulted in transforming these previously experienced private concerns into public issues (Gabe and Bury 1988, 1991a; Gabe et al. 1991). In this context, mass media have emerged as key definers of the language of dependency and have offered a redefinition of 'normal' drug use. Within these public discussions a heightened awareness and willingness of individuals to talk about their dependency have been the results.

As women have entered the labour market in growing numbers over the past two decades, the changes in women's role in society have led to speculation about how women's working role will alter their health habits and health status (Verbrugge 1989). In the area of alcohol research, the so-called *convergence hypothesis* was used in the early 1980s as a predictive statement. This hypothesis postulates that women's employment in the labour market will change their social position in such a way that the traditional female role will give way to behaviours previously pursued by men. The assumption here is that women will increase their alcohol consumption as part of their participation in the public sphere (Ferrence 1980).

Psychotropic drug researchers (Ferrence and Whitehead 1980) have proposed that, as women's alcohol use increases, their use of psychotropics will diminish. Hence, the substitution hypothesis would appear to explain also working women's orientations towards alcohol and psychotropics. Yet, the convergence hypothesis was not confirmed in North American studies carried out in the 1970s (Ferrence 1980; Ferrence and Whitehead 1980). National surveys in the Nordic countries show that women's drinking increased in the 1970s and 1980s. But women still drink a small fraction of men's consumption (Järvinen and Olafsdottir 1989). Furthermore, women's problem drinking in the Nordic countries is much less frequent than men's and 'never took on the same ritualistic nature as men's' (Salmose 1989:42). The substitution hypothesis has not been confirmed, given that women's use of psychotropics has not declined proportionately – either in relation to their alcohol use or their labour market participation.

As we can see, the convergence hypothesis has been confirmed only partially in the case of women. Although changes have occurred in women's drinking habits, their double rate of consumption of psychotropics has, however, remained unchanged during the same period. Furthermore, the substitution hypothesis does not provide an accurate picture of women's attitudes towards drugs and alcohol in today's context, although to our knowledge this hypothesis has never been empirically tested for either gender. Nevertheless, this hypothesis is a taken-for-granted fact when men's use of psychotropics is described.

In sum, many of the above discussions, both the 'women-are-expressive' hypothesis and the substitution hypothesis, are based on a functionalist perspective. However, the 'women-are-expressive' hypothesis focuses only on women's illness behaviour and relates this behaviour to the female role in society. Hence, a high rate of psychotropic drug use among women is explained by their emotionality, viewed as part of their female role. In this way, women's health problems are seen to exist within women's biology rather than being related to key structural factors implicit within the prevailing class or gender system. The result of this view is that women's use of psychotropics tends to be trivialised because this use is assumed to reflect merely 'normal' differences between men and women. Ultimately, this conceptualisation process reinforces the notion that women are destined by biology, a taken-for-granted fact of 'nature'.

We saw that the substitution hypothesis addresses the issue of why men use psychotropics less often than women. The tacit functionalist argument is that women's and men's use of relaxation-producing substances is related to gender-specific norms. The assumption is that men self-medicate their anxieties by using alcohol and, therefore, do not need psychotropics. On the other hand, the proponents of this hypothesis do not state whether alcohol has merely a preventive function, or whether its use has similar medical effects on the same symptoms that women treat with psychotropics. The narrow focus on psychotropic drugs as a specific female attribute has limited further explorations of key issues. For example, this type of focus has neglected explanations concerning the high rate of psychotropic drug use among certain subgroups of men as well as the apparently increasing dual dependency problem – the combined use of alcohol and psychotropics – among men.

Structural perspectives on psychotropic drug use

A major theme of classical sociology is the increasing globalisation and differentiation of society, a fragmentation process splitting society into various unequal groups. The Weberian account describes this process in terms of the emergence of status groups, while the Marxist account portrays this process as the emergence of two distinct social classes. Both accounts result in a structural materialist perspective on health and illness – a perspective viewing people's location in the socio-economic system as a key to determining their health. The contingent characteristics according to a Weberian account are, for example, occupation, gender, race, ethnicity and religion, while within a Marxist account class, as defined by the specific mode of production in society, is the chief analytical site.

Nevertheless, survey research on psychotropic drug use, which attempts to operationalise a Weberian structural perspective, has identified gender as being the most important contingent characteristic. Simply, women use psychotropics twice as often as men. Furthermore, age has also been found to be a crucial explanatory factor in the use of all types of drug as well as in the specific case of psychotropics (Cooperstock and Parnell 1982). Race and income appear as other contingent factors related to the use of psychotropics. Let us take a closer look at these two contingent factors: race and income.

Black people have been observed to have much lower rates of psychotropic drug use than white people in the United States (Cafferata and Kasper 1983; Wells *et al*. 1985) and Britain (Gabe and Thorogood 1986). Gabe and Thorogood have shown, in their study of black and white working-class women in London, that long-term use of psychotropics was situationally determined. The meaning of and the perceived need for psychotropics were related to the extent of social integration of these two racial groups. White women were more loosely integrated into the local social structure than black women. Hence, white women were more often long-term users of psychotropics. Other studies on women's use of psychotropics have pointed out the importance of social networks and social support systems as explanatory factors (e.g. Cafferata *et al*. 1983).

Focusing on income, early survey studies revealed that the use of psychotropics was more prevalent among higher- than lower-income groups (e.g. Parry 1968; Pflanz *et al*. 1977). In contrast, later studies have documented a higher prevalence of use among lower-income or socio-economic groups than higher ones (e.g. Bakka *et al*. 1974; Jartsell and Nordegren 1976; Cafferata and Kasper 1983; Riska and Klaukka 1984; Isacson and Haglund 1988; Ashton and Golding 1989). Most of these studies have noted simply the prevalence of use. Their authors have omitted placing key social characteristics such as income or socio-economic status in a theoretical framework which would help to explain variations. The emergent social characteristics appear to represent a shared structural position, defining an individual's access to material and social resources in society.

In discussing structural perspectives on psychotropic drug use, we flag up briefly the Marxist account – an account of ill health which relates the distribution of ill health to the location of individuals within the class structure (Navarro 1976). However, this kind of explanation has not surfaced in the literature on psychotropic drug use as has the above Weberian account. Chapter 4 will provide an overview of the Marxist perspective as applied to an analysis of psychotropic drug use.

The social constructionist perspective

The social constructionist perspective sees social phenomena as a product of a social process in which social actors attach meanings to and define the world around them. Likewise, health and illness are not inherent in any behaviour or condition, but rather products of social definitions of normal or expected behaviours in certain social contexts. Thus, illness and mental health are not biologically given states, but embedded in social relations and, as such, relative, socially defined or constructed phenomena. In this context, the labelling approach to mental health, along with its (at the time) innovative conceptual framework (e.g. Scheff 1966; Goffman 1961), preceded discussions on the notion of medical discourse which has emerged within current sociological debates on postmodernism (Rosenau 1992; Fox 1993). Recently, the work of Michel Foucault (1975) has inspired sociologists to interpret critically developments in public health and community medicine (Armstrong 1983) and the social perceptions of the body (Turner 1984, 1992; Frank 1990; Daly 1990; Martin 1989; Butler 1993; Shilling 1993) from a social constructionist perspective.

In psychotropic drug research, the social constructionist view has been advanced mainly in British studies. Two major themes appear in these studies. The first is the social and symbolic meaning that users of psychotropic drugs attach to their use (e.g. Helman 1981; Gabe and Thorogood 1986). In these studies, the social meaning of tranquilliser use has been viewed as *the* central feature explaining the extent of and the dependency on tranquilliser use.

The second theme apparent in the social constructionist accounts of psychotropics is the role exerted by the mass media in constructing representations of the normal versus the problem psychotropic drug user. In this setting, the 'normal' user is constructed in the advertisements for psychotropic drugs in medical journals. While these advertisements do not target the patients directly, they are aimed at prescribing physicians. Therefore, these advertising strategies differ slightly from those which appeal directly to the potential consumer of a product. Here it must be remembered that physicians act as a gatekeeping mechanism in the legal acquisition of psychotropics. Hence, the strategies used in psychotropic drug advertisements reveal not only stereo-typical pictures of patients but also metaphors in order to influence physicians' prescribing patterns (Chapman 1979; Goldman and Montagne 1986; Montagne 1988; Neill 1989). With regard to the latter strategy, metaphors assist the viewer (the physician) to attach a certain symbolic meaning to each drug advertised. Therefore, these drug metaphors have a powerful influence on physicians' prescribing habits. A further detailed discussion on metaphors as well as a presentation on trends in drug advertising with special refer-ence to psychotropic drugs will be presented in Chapter 5.

In addition to studies examining the cultural representa-tions of the 'normal' user portrayed in psychotropic drug ad-vertising, there have been studies on how the mass media have influenced the definition of the 'problem' user. Gabe and Bury (1991b; Gabe *et al.* 1991) have examined British television programmes which were produced in the 1980s and which covered critically the extent of use and dependency on tranquillisers. These authors highlight the images and narrative structure utilised in this discursive, media coverage on tranquilliser use. The imagery suggests that tranquillisers are frightening and addictive drugs. Furthermore, these drugs have the potential to make innocent British subjects 'addictive victims'. On the other hand, implicit within the narrative structure are the emotional and symbolic meanings of tranquilliser use and dependency. In this context, two major pairs of actors appear in this television coverage: one pair is the innocent consumer versus the drug-prescribing physician, while the other pair is the ordinary general practitioner versus the more clinically oriented specialist. Gabe and Bury contend that a crisis of confidence in the physician–patient relationship, as well as a deep questioning of the role of medical treatments, emerge as key issues in this media scenario.

As can be seen from the above discussions, the social constructionist perspective has been the dominant approach in studies, examining not only the specific, symbolic or social meaning of psychotropics for users but also the role of the mass media in structuring the cultural representations of users.

Overall implications of user-oriented perspectives

From a sociological as well as a feminist perspective, the user-oriented perspective is fraught with contradictions. On the positive side, this perspective has turned attention away from the view that drug use is somehow related to individual pathology to a fuller view in which characteristics of key groups are able to emerge. Hence, social factors external to individuals become visible. On the negative side, an individualised notion of use has been the outcome of this genre of studies. This remains a paradox. As we indicated in Chapters 1 and 2, the reason for this paradox lies in the character of the data in studies on users. These studies are based on surveys, which provide a cross-sectional picture of the general population or a population group. Scant information exists on the structures mediating between the individual user and the health care system as well as on the complex process whereby a user is introduced to, terminates or continues psychotropic drug use. Thus, the reasons for psychotropic drug use are given either an individualistic or a voluntaristic interpretation. The individualistic interpretation depicts use in a deterministic way, a behavioural outcome of certain individual attributes, such as income, sex, education and so on. The voluntaristic interpretation, on the other hand, portrays the user as a social actor who has identified by himself or herself a need for drug therapy and, in turn, has decided to seek medical assistance for his or her symptoms. The voluntaristic approach conveys a view of the user as overtly rational: he or she decides to seek professional help in order to relieve symptoms of distress. Here, drug use is perceived as being based on the user's own decision and choice of action. Regardless of its emphasis on rationality, the voluntaristic approach portrays users as acting in a social vacuum where other social actors, such as significant others and physicians, are made invisible.

PROVIDER-ORIENTED PERSPECTIVES

Physician characteristics

Let us now turn our attention to provider-oriented perspectives. The user of psychotropics is not a consumer in the traditional sense of the word. In fact, 'consumer choice' refers more to the prescribing physician than the patient/user. Consumer behaviour which is otherwise encouraged on the more general, commercial market is not supported on the more specific medical market. Hence, 'doctor shopping' is a term with negative connotations in the case of psychotropics. 'Doctor shopping' is used more in relationship to the abuse of psychotropic drugs than a user's rational consumer behaviour.

Studies that focus on providers of psychotropics take the stance that it is the physician who makes the drug choice for the patient. The latter complies; buys the prescribed drug from a pharmacy; and uses the drug according to the prescribed dose. Within the context of these studies, explanations for drug use can be found in the physician's choice of drug regimen rather than the user's behaviour. Here, the physician's choice has been related to the type of medical practice as well as the type of information received about these drugs (Hemminki 1975). Early studies with this focus were concerned about excessive prescribing of benzodiazepines by general practitioners (Parish 1971; Raynes 1979; Petursson and Lader 1981) and the influence of physician characteristics on attitudes towards the legitimate use of psychotropic drugs

(Linn 1971). In this area, a recent longitudinal study of prescriptions for psychotropic medications in the United States revealed a decreasing role for the primary care physician as a provider of psychotropics (Olfson and Klerman 1993:561). This study showed that the proportion of psychotropic drug visits to primary care physicians decreased from 64 per cent in 1980 to 55 per cent in 1985, and 52 per cent in 1989. During this same nine-year period, the proportion of psychotropic drug visits to psychiatrists increased from 15 per cent to 25 per cent. In a related context, a recent Swedish prescription study found that physicians, both within internal medicine and psychiatry, chose more high-dosage (what the authors term high-quantity) prescriptions than physicians in other specialties (Isacson *et al.* 1993:345–7).

In short, a number of studies of psychotropic drug use have focused primarily on physicians' characteristics as being the main explanation for a user's initiation and continuation of drug use. Studies which have used a feminist framework also fall within this genre. Feminists have pointed to male dominance within the medical profession; the inherent sexism in medical practice; and the gendering of drug prescribing as an explanation of women's over-representation among users (Fisher 1986; Ettorre 1992). Other studies have shown that women are provided with psychotropics controlling for symptoms more often than men. A study based on an analysis of data from the 1985 National Ambulatory Medical Care Survey in the United States (Hohmann 1989) showed that, in comparison to men, women presenting the same complaints, psychiatric diagnoses, symptom diagnoses, interactive states as well as demographic and health services characteristics were significantly more likely than men to receive prescriptions for tranquillisers and antidepressants, but not hypnotics, barbiturates or neuroleptics. In this work, Hohmann notes that physicians did not interpret men's alcohol problems as a sign of mental disorder capable of alleviation by psychotropics. In this area, cautious prescribing behaviour has been raised as an issue owing to the emergence of a dual dependency problem, especially for men – an issue noted earlier.

In a related context, a Nordic study based on self-reported

drug use and the presence of psychiatric symptomatology showed that, in comparison to Danish men, Danish women reported more frequently the use of hypnotics-sedatives controlling for symptomatology, while in Finland this gender pattern was found to be reversed (Riska *et al.* 1993:57). Also, there were no gender differences controlling for symptomatology in the self-reported use of tranquillisers in both countries.

Pharmaceutical industry

Historically, drug companies as providers of psychotropics have introduced new drugs on the medical market continuously, while physicians have generally been dependent on commercial sources for information about new drugs (Hemminki 1975). The role of advertising and drug retailing in the dissemination of drug information has been viewed primarily as a mechanism of market expansion (Lexchin 1987, 1989, 1994). Here, the drug promotion strategies of pharmaceutical companies have been criticised because they tend to emphasise irrelevant aspects rather than pharmacological facts about these drugs. Hence, physicians' decisions about drug therapy appear to be related more to the commercial efforts of drug companies than to independent, medical decisions, based on scientific knowledge (Avorn *et al.* 1982; Krupka and Vener 1985). Research has shown that commercial rather than medical sources are more important for general practitioners when prescribing a new drug, while specialists receive this information from medical sources (Peay and Peay 1988, 1990).

As we have seen, the provider perspective, which focuses on the pharmaceutical industry as the generator of psychotropic drug sales, considers both the physician and the drug user as mere objects of the profit-making motive of the drug industry. Neither the physician nor the patient is seen as an independent decision maker. The primary agent is this industry which, in order to maximise profits, is seen to work through both the physician and the patient.

In conclusion, by analysing previous works on psychotropic drug use through a sociological lens, we have shown that this type of research has a dualistic character – it focuses either on the user or the provider. We have suggested that this orientation results in an overemphasis on the endeavours of one actor to the exclusion of the other. At the same time, this orientation renders invisible other social actors involved in this complex process which results in psychotropic drug use. Current theoretical perspectives have tended to address the motives or structures guiding either the user or the provider. We contend that by making visible the various types of actor, as well as the activities they engage in at various social and cultural levels, one acquires a clearer understanding of how drug use is socially constructed. In this context, there is a need for building a framework in which this type of visibility and understanding are ensured. Furthermore, if we want to understand the experiences of sufferers, we need to appreciate the gendered character of psychotropic drug use as an increasingly visible form of health and social behaviour. These issues will be discussed in the next chapter when we look at the emergent layers of analyses which need to be examined for a comprehensive view of the workings of this behaviour.

Chapter 4

Making gender visible
Seeing 'layers' in the social construction of psychotropic drug use

TRADITIONAL SOCIOLOGICAL PERSPECTIVES ON PSYCHOTROPIC DRUG USE: PROBLEMS, DEFINITIONS AND SOLUTIONS

In the previous chapters, our contention has been that much of the research on psychotropic drug use either has an untheoretical character or harbours a theoretical approach, based on hidden assumptions in the research framework. To ease the reader's understanding, we will, in this chapter, attempt to unfold these assumptions and subsequently locate them within the major, existing sociological perspectives. For heuristic purposes, we present a brief review of the traditional sociological perspectives on health and drug behaviour and offer a critique of their shortcomings from a feminist perspective. We will then construct our own theoretical framework which not only represents a social constructionist approach to psychotropic drug use but also highlights the various social actors and emergent layers evident in the construction of psychotropic drug use.

Three major sociological perspectives can be used to explain psychotropic drug use: the functionalist, the Marxist and the symbolic interactionist. In reviewing these perspectives, four questions and respective dimensions can be considered:

1 What is conceptualised as the major problem with regard to psychotropic drug use? (the conceptual dimension)
2 What kind of intervention is proposed to solve this problem? (the instrumental dimension)

3 What appears as the desired outcome of the recommended intervention? (the eventual dimension)
4 What is conceptualised as the optimum state? (the adaptational dimension)

Let us look at the implications of the above considerations. According to the proponents of a functionalist perspective, the major problem is conceptualised as a deficient role performance owing to ill health. In the case of anxiety or insomnia, the most expedient solution is a prescription for psychotropics, most often tranquillisers or sleeping-pills. It is therefore thought that this drug regimen will restore the user to optimum role performance. In this sense, drug use has a system-maintenance function: the user adapts, while the drug is viewed as instrumental in this adaptation process.

Within a Marxist perspective, the prevailing class system is a direct reflection of the capitalist mode of production. Any person's well-being, both materially and in terms of health, is a product of his or her own location within the class structure (Navarro 1976). The picture, here, is one in which any significant improvements in the health status of the subordinated classes in society, including women, can be achieved only by a total and radical redistribution of income and wealth in society (Fee 1983). Psychotropic drugs are, in this sense, an 'opiate' for the masses: they individualise illness and conceal the class-determinated character of illnesses. (Interestingly enough, this term has been appropriated by the medical profession, see Lader 1978.) A radical change of the exploitative features inherent in the capitalist mode of production and, in turn, the enhancement of social equality will eliminate the existence of 'problem populations' or what the Marxist representatives have called the 'raw material' for 'deviance production' (Spitzer 1975:642).

Proponents of both the functionalist and Marxist perspectives view the development of specialised control systems as an integral part of modern society. This type of system analysis, inherent in both perspectives, implies that the medical profession is the main agent in controlling the kind of deviancy which is subsumed under the label illness. In this specific sense, psychotropics appear as a form of social control, sustaining the existing social order (Koumjian 1981). This form of chemical dependency appears to uphold society's orderly currents.

On the other hand, the symbolic interactionist perspective is based on an agency analysis of deviance and social control. Deviancy is a label imposed on subjects who, in their rejection or acceptance of these labels, construct deviant identities and careers. A radical transformation can be accomplished only by challenging and rebuilding the existing 'hierarchy of credibility' (Becker 1967). The outcome is a renegotiation of normality; a major shift in the ethical basis for deviant definitions; and the establishment of new moral codes within society.

In the light of this discussion, a gender-sensitive perspective challenges the invisibility of gender in both the system and agency analyses, evident in the above perspectives. It does this in three ways. First, it challenges the functionalists by pointing to the primacy they give to normative factors in explaining social phenomena. In Parsons' writing, gender is recognised in the private sphere of social relations, whereas market relations are assumed to be guided by universalistic (i.e. gender-neutral) criteria. Here, gender is merely a particularistic (and *not* patriarchal) criterion which will wither away with the increasing rationalisation of society.

Second, a gender perspective challenges the overdetermined view of social inequality, implicit in Marxist thinking. Marxist theorists see the economic system or the sphere of production as being the primary divider of people into social categories (i.e. classes), and women, as appendages to men, are *primarily* members of social classes. The focus is on the capitalist economy, which produces social inequality and related social problems, and not on gender inequality. Feminist theorists have criticised this somewhat overwhelming emphasis on economic structures and classes explicit within Marxist theory. Instead, they point to reproduction and patriarchy as the primary generators of social inequality. Thus, they emphasise a focus on the complex, social divisions (including class and race) between men and women (Walby 1990:11; Maynard 1990:277).

Third, a gender-sensitive perspective challenges the

symbolic interactionists' focus on agency analyses because they do not recognise men as *the* 'moral entrepreneurs' and as the more powerful (*vis-à-vis* women) constructors of discourses and moral codes. This type of analysis is gender neutral. With reference to our specific topic, psychotropic drug use, there is a need, therefore, to address the gendered character of medical and/or 'deviant' labels attributed to symptoms and diagnoses as well as the gendered criteria utilised in medical decision making. Hence, we note again our contention that gender differences in psychotropic drug use are *concrete* manifestations of an underlying structure – the social institution of gender (Lorber 1994:7). Furthermore, we maintain that an understanding of the gendered process by which psychotropic drug use is socially constructed, produced and reproduced is achieved by 'unpacking' and thereby illuminating the intricate layers explicit in this process.

LAYERS IN THE SOCIAL CONSTRUCTION OF PSYCHOTROPIC DRUG USE

In order to set the scene for our discussion on layers in the social construction of psychotropic drug use, let us first turn our attention briefly to the two discursive accounts generally referred to in the literature: those presented by lay people and by the physician. Medical diagnosis – whether lay or professional – is an interpretative process through which illnesses and diseases are constructed. Every culture has its codes for translating signs into symptoms; for linking symptomatologies to etiologies and interventions; for confirming translations; and for legitimising interventions (Law 1985:187). Focusing on the codes confirmed in this translation process is especially important when examining expressions of distress and disorder. Law (1985:187) identifies three levels of cultural interpretation of disease in research on folk idioms for emotional distress. The first level is that symptoms are culturally expressed through the body as a symbol system. The second is that symptoms are culturally received, sorted and identified within both the prevailing theory of disease and the cultural rules of etiology. The process in which symptoms are given socio-cultural meanings, based on the value hierarchy of

a specific local, social context, comprises the third interpretative level.

Historically, the notion of women's 'nerves' has been a lay
metaphor for defining women's emotional and physical
condition *vis-à-vis* men's (Davis and Whitten 1988; Chesler
1989). Today, the notion of 'nerves' as a lay or folk idiom for
anxiety and depression (Nations *et al.* 1988) is assumed to exist
primarily in traditional societies. On the other hand, in
modern society, 'nerves as a folk idiom' is assumed to come
under the purview of the medical profession: physicians
diagnose and treat 'it'.

In this context, we challenge this dualistic notion of traditional versus professional definitions of symptoms on two
grounds. First, individuals do not live in a social and cultural
vacuum. Rather, in their everyday lives, men and women
attempt to make sense of the world around them and their
location within it. They interact in this social world through
their bodies – their working bodies, their gendered bodies.
Significantly, conflicts between their perceived selves and
their physical and social surroundings are awarded a symptomatic expression. Within this interactive process, a dialogue of
symptoms' meanings is created by the actors involved – the
individual, friends and family, and the professional – through
interpretative frameworks. Mutually supportive, or competing, discursive accounts are provided in this interactive
process. Nevertheless, these accounts coalesce, forming the
medical discourse, which, in turn, transforms self-defined
symptoms into a representation of illness. In contemporary
society, the lay, traditional discourse proceeds from the
professional medical discourse, based on scientific knowledge.
Therefore, constructing symptoms of ill health involves a
'discursive mixture' of definitions from both discourses.

Second, *all* severe symptoms are not presented to the
professional; rather, these symptoms remain within the lay
culture of healing. Specifically, not all symptoms of anxiety
and depression are recognised and treated. One American
study found that only 27 per cent of primary practitioners
working in an ambulatory practice diagnosed correctly
anxiety and depression. Interestingly enough, these states
were presented in lay culture or folk terms as 'nerves' (Nations

et al. 1988:1245). Similarly, expressions of distress, which appear more frequently among men than women (e.g. substance abuse problems, outbreaks of violence) are not generally associated with mental health problems as is women's display of depression (Pugliesi 1992:55).

Hence, we contend that an understanding of the initiation, continuation and termination of psychotropic drug use demands an analysis of the various levels whereby cultural interpretations of symptoms, illness and diseases are constructed and legitimised. In our view, there are five primary actors involved in the dialogue whereby psychotropic drug use is socially constructed:

1 the individual
2 groups
3 the medical profession
4 the pharmaceutical industry
5 the health care system.

The behaviour of these actors can be conceptualised at three different levels:

1 the way the actor expresses or reacts to a need for psychotropics;
2 the way the actor behaves as a response to this need; and
3 the cognitive dimension which constructs and legitimises this need.

Table 4.1 outlines actors' major endeavours along the suggested three dimensions of activity: the expressive, behavioural and cognitive dimensions.

Within this scheme, let us look at the first actor. The *individual* perceives a variety of vague symptoms which are interpreted through the cultural codes available for bodily symptoms. He or she begins a 'narrative construction'. In the words of Williams (1984:178), a *narrative* is a 'process of continous accounting whereby the mundane incidents and events of daily life are given some kind of plausible order'. Hence, the individual interprets the symptoms first as routine 'everyday problems', but if these symptoms persist and form a more well-defined character, a 'casual exploring of diagnosis' will construct the symptoms as stress. Here, the notion of

Table 4.1 Layers in the social construction of psychotropic drug use

Actor	Expression	Behaviour	Cognitive dimension
Individual	Self-perceived symptoms	Role strains	Personal narratives
Groups	Gendered moods: stress, nerves	Lay referral	Lay culture and idioms
Medical profession	Medical diagnosis: prescription	Legitimation of the sick role through drug prescription	Medical gaze
Pharmaceutical companies	Market	Sales	Advertising
Health care system	Prevalence of psychotropic drug use. Prescription rates	Regulation of supply and demand	Epidemiological gaze

'stress' carries a wide array of socio-cultural meanings. Within the context of lay culture, the most common etiology provided for the more medically known 'breakdowns' of a body's normal functioning is stress. In Blaxter's (1983:64) study of Scottish women's experiences of ill health, stress and strains were the most popular categories for the cause of disease. Nevertheless, the women studied resented doctors' attempts to impose similar explanations on their illness experiences. In this context, Williams' (1984:178) study on the narrative reconstruction of the genesis of chronic illness shows that there are gender differences in the perception of the characteristics of stressors. On the one hand, Bill, the male studied by Williams, referred to sources external to himself – his work – as the reason for his illness. On the other hand, Gill, the woman, interpreted her illness within the framework of internal causation. She noted an 'internal psychological pathology'. Here, the discourse on stress can be seen to construct the medical meaning of external and internal stressors, leading to pathological consequences for individuals – but in a gendered way. Furthermore, when individuals provide accounts of their perceptions of their own health to families, friends or physicians, *personal narratives* constitute a major source of information. By providing a personal narrative, an individual not only structures his or her self-perceived symptoms but also places the actual nature of his or her illness in a temporal as well as a gendered context. A further discussion of this concept will be presented in Chapter 6.

The second 'actor' contributing to the dialogue on psychotropic drug use is the *group*. At this level, personal narratives are received and interpreted by others initially as 'stress', a lay idiom for both the cause and experience of minor psychiatric symptomatology. The lay culture has a variety of responses, depending on the class, age, ethnicity, race and gender of the 'sufferer' involved. A lay referral system proposes a set of structured actions to restore the sufferer's health and well-being through the use of non-professional advice and remedies. Suggested actions may include a whole stream of 'lay advice', but suggestions inevitably are attempts to help ameliorate everyday stresses. For example, 'take a drink', 'take a walk', 'eat a good meal', 'increase exercise', 'enrol in a yoga class' or 'join a self-help group'. Lay measures may also include a sharing of psychotropics with someone who complains about his or her symptoms. If the symptoms persist, encouragement to see a doctor may be a suggested measure. Nevertheless, lay measures may also be received and given throughout the entire course of an illness.

The third actor is the *medical profession*. Physicians listen to the personal narratives of their patients and use this information as a basis for diagnosis and medical decision making (see Kleinman 1988; Waitzkin 1991). In a concrete sense, the 'medical gaze' guides the physician in this translation process from signs, symptoms, etiologies to interventions. The prevailing medical discourse – biomedicine – provides a cognitive map for interpreting as well as defining the patient's narrative and physical symptoms into medically recognised categories. Depending on the severity of the symptoms, the sick role is either awarded temporarily by the physician or reflects a chronic state. At the very least, a medical label mixes with a sick role. In this context, prescribing psychotropics appears clearly within the social space where physicians bestow and legitimate medical labels for specific symptoms or conditions. Physicians' definitions of certain human behaviours in medical terms tend to reduce the moral meaning of these respective behaviours. Simply, physicians' definitions may have the power to raise various illness behaviours, including 'nerves', to levels of social acceptability. Although legal psychotropic drug use may be viewed as socially acceptable behaviour, important questions remain unanswered. Why do some groups of long-term users conceal their psychotropic drug use from others? Why do negative feelings emerge? For example, on the one hand, physicians' definitions of psychotropic drug use may objectively raise 'nerves' to a respectable level. On the other hand, there is a distinct aura of unacceptability attached to this process on a subjective level. Indeed, negativity, extreme fear and deep depression can be seen to surface when reviewing literature – particularly literature reflecting female users' points of view (Jerome 1991; Trickett 1991; Haddon 1984; Curran and Golombok 1985; Melville 1984). As Jerome aptly states:

> Once you've been prescribed benzodiazepines you may be labelled as someone who needs drugs to sleep, or as unable to cope with your life. . . . You are more at risk of being given other mood-altering drugs on another occasion than someone who hasn't had tranquillisers. . . . When the GP gives you a prescription . . . he may also write down in your medical history that you are suffering with nerves, neurotic or have a personality disorder. That label always hangs over you.
>
> (Jerome 1991:27)

In short, the process of reducing moral meaning on the part of the physician may be, in the case of psychotropic drug prescribing, a discriminating process which is gender based.

The fourth actor involved in this dialogue is the *pharmaceutical industry*. It acts on the commercial market, where sales of its products, drugs, are a measure of success. Advertising in medical journals is the main channel to promote its products. In this context, advertisements for prescribed drugs are rarely, if ever, read by the potential or actual consumer of the drugs. Therefore, while advertisements are addressed primarily to the prescribing physician, they must be presented in a way which appeals to the physician. Ultimately, advertisements aim to influence any physician's inclination to choose a certain brand among other competing brands on the medical market. But advertisements reveal also how certain definitions and meanings of psychotropic drug use are constructed. In effect, advertisements are representations and specific expressions of the medical discourse, promoted by the pharmaceutical industry.

We identify the *health care system* as the fifth actor in the dialogue on psychotropic drugs, while a variety of agencies within it monitor the drug market. Researchers make visible the prevalence of psychotropic drug use by means of surveys. Studies in clinical settings provide information about the dependency-producing effects of long-term use of these drugs. National health authorities advise on prescription rates and sales. For example, the Nordic countries have a joint medical council which gathers annual sales statistics on the use of prescribed medications. Advertisements for both over-the-counter and prescribed medicines in the Nordic countries are controlled by public authorities. Since prescribed medicines are either subsidised purchases or free of charge (i.e. as part of the national sickness insurance system) specific control policies on the sales of drugs are part of national health policy in the Nordic setting. In examining the Canadian marketing codes, Lexchin (1994) suggests that, even if codes for controlling pharmaceutical promotion exist, there are difficulties in sanctioning those companies that violate them.

Concern over excess use of psychotropics or over-prescribing may result in a change in a nation's drug policy. For example, a dramatic drop in the sales of hypnotics-sedatives between 1986 and 1987 in Iceland has been explained by a revision in prescription rules. A national policy endorsed the enforcement of smaller dosages (Hansen and Gyldmark 1990: 201–2). Another example is the concern over the effects of triazolam, sold worldwide as Halcion. This concern resulted in the temporary withdrawal of that drug from the commercial market in a number of Western countries.

The cognitive dimensions of the health care system can be called the 'epidemiological gaze' (Armstrong 1983:10). This gaze can further be identified as a way of seeing use and problem use (i.e. abuse, misuse) of psychotropics in the general population. In this context, intervention strategies consist of a variety of regulatory measures used to influence the supply and demand of psychotropics. For example, regulations can be directed towards the medical profession in the form of changes in the recommended duration and levels of dosages in prescriptions for certain psychotropics. Regulations can be directed towards the distributive mechanism utilised by local pharmacies or multinational drug companies. Most strikingly, regulations can include the withdrawal of a particular drug from the market. Nevertheless, there is scant research evaluating the implications of regulatory measures. To label high rates of tranquilliser use as a 'social problem' and to withdraw certain tranquillisers from the market do not solve problems at the individual, subjective level. Faced with increasing negative labels of drug use or more stringent regulation of psychoactive substances, individuals construct alternative routes of supply or drug innovations. These respective routes and innovations can be developed within the health care system as a way of securing a concealed access to drugs. While the hidden structure of drug provision has been explored thoroughly in research on illegal drugs, the hidden structure of psychotropic drug provision, which remains within as well as beyond the boundaries of the health care system, is less known.

THE LAYERED STRUCTURE OF PSYCHOTROPICS: IMPLICATIONS FOR WOMEN

Now that we have examined the intricacies involved in the social construction of psychotropic drug use, let us focus our attention on how this process affects women. Recently, a number of feminist health scholars have pointed to women's bodies as being primary targets in the expansion of medicine. This genre of literature has shown that women's normal bodily functions have been defined as pathological. They appear as functions to be controlled by professionals, i.e. the medical profession. The term 'medicalisation' has been used as a broad concept to describe the annexation of the human body under the legitimate supervision and control of the medical profession (Conrad 1992). More recently, a number of scholars (Riessman 1992; Theriot 1993) have contended, however, that not only have women been passive objects in this process but also that middle-class women, in particular, have actively participated in the construction of new medical definitions. In this context, the 'victimisation perspective' is challenged by Theriot. Her account places women's voices in medical discourses as both patients and physicians. The latter group were embroiled in arguments, based on competing professional interests of male gynaecologists, neurologists and alienists/psychiatrists concerning the etiology of women's illness in nineteenth-century American society. Theriot demonstrates how women physicians supported the existing neurological and psychiatric viewpoint as opposed to the gynaecological one, which tied women's nervousness and mental illness to female reproductive organs (Theriot 1993:12–13). The latter viewpoint – a form of 'gynaecological essentialism' – was, however, embraced by the patients and their families as an interpretation of the etiology of women's distress.

Martin's (1989) study of American middle-class and working-class women's views of their reproductive functions revealed that middle-class women embraced a reductionistic view, explicit within the biomedical discourse, while working-class women preferred a holistic view of the healthy functioning of their bodies. Similarly, Calnan (1988; Calnan and Williams 1992:240), in a study of lay views on scientific medicine, found that, in comparison to middle-class women, working-class women were more negative towards doctors' prescribing of tranquillisers. Middle-class women appeared to be more positive or ambivalent. Calnan (1988) suggests that middle-class more than working-class women's faith in scientific medicine is related to the symmetry between modern medicine and the cultural orientation of the middle class. In Calnan's view, medical ideology is congruent with bourgeois ideology.

In effect, Riessman, Theriot, Martin and Calnan propose that the class interests of middle-class women have made them more prone than working-class women to be assimilated into the medical paradigm, upheld by the male-dominated medical profession. Within this interpretation, working-class women emerge as the victors rather than the victims (as is the case in traditional Marxist approaches). Working-class women's traditionalised, lay approach to medicine is portrayed as providing them with a shield of independence. They become the bearers of the 'pure' health culture for women. This essentialist notion of working-class women's health culture is contrasted with the subordinated status of middle-class women, lumbered with a medical discourse which reduces their female bodies to objects.

The merit of the above interpretation is that it points to the *diversity of women*. Differences among women can be used as an analytical site. However, the above interpretation provides an over-glorified notion of working-class women and their apparent independent relationship to modern medicine. Statistics tend to show that, in comparison to middle-class women, working-class women use various health services more frequently. As Calnan (1988) correctly ponders, working-class women's scepticism of modern medicine may, in fact, be related to their experiences of discrimination and inferior care provided in health facilities to which they have had access. In reality, middle-class women have been in the forefront of public health debates focused on women's issues. These women have mobilised efforts to reclaim not only knowledge about, but also ownership and treatment of, their own bodies. Within the context of developments in the new reproductive technologies, female ownership of female bodies has emerged as a key issue of concern. In the 1970s, the women's health movements, both in the United States and Britain, began the arduous work of reclaiming women's collective knowledge of their bodies (Ruzek 1976; Doyal 1983; Mellow 1989). Noticeably, this was primarily a middle-class movement. Current initiatives among American women physicians to establish a specialty in women's health reflects efforts aimed at providing a type of feminised health care – where women are at the centre of the knowledge and practice of health service provisions (Johnson and Dawson 1990). Both the women's health movement and this recent professional project to create a specialty in women's health have been led by middle-class women. But there is an absence of working-class women as visible actors within these endeavours.

Following on from the above discussion, we contend that full conceptualisations of the *individual* and *group* levels of analysis in the social construction of psychotropic drug use must recognise the diversity of women. Class, race, age, sexual preference, ethnicity and being able-bodied are key factors that can provide a broader structural and cultural context for interpretations and expressions of symptoms. In a related context, Chapter 6 focuses on the individual level of analysis and provides examples of the personal narratives of women and men concerning their psychotropic drug use. Gender differences in the functions of the lay referral system for these users will be discussed in Chapter 7, which explores the group level of analysis.

Moving on to the next level of analysis, we see that through the prevailing biomedical discourse the *medical profession* constructs women's symptoms into medical categories. As Riessman (1992:114) has pointed out: 'Medicalization has resulted in the construction of medical meanings of *normal* functions in women. . . . By contrast, routine experiences that are uniquely male remain largely unstudied by medical science and, consequently, are rarely treated by physicians as potentially pathological.' The medicalisation of women's symptoms was also pointed out in Cooperstock's (1971) classic article on gender differences in psychotropic drug use. In that context, Cooperstock asserted that the cultural beliefs of male physicians rendered them more likely to assign psychiatric labels to women's than men's emotional distress and, hence, to prescribe drugs to this assigned group: women. As women are entering the medical profession in increasing numbers, optimistic voices have expressed the view that sexist labels and the treatment of women's ill health will wither away (Altekruse and McDermott 1987:85; Miles 1991). Nevertheless, there is thus far no convincing empirical evidence to support unequivocally that contention. While women physicians have been shown to be more empathic towards patients, they do not differ dramatically from their male colleagues in diagnosis or therapy choices (Riska and Wegar 1995).

In the 1970s, *pharmaceutical companies* displayed mainly women in their advertisements for psychotropics. At the same time, advertisements for other drugs had a more even gender distribution or at least portrayed men more often than women in psychotropics advertisements (Mant and Darroch 1975; Prather and Fidell 1975). Since the end of the 1970s, a new trend in drug advertising has been documented. Advertisements have become more gender neutral. If there is a person in the advertisement, it is more frequently a man than a woman (Thompson 1979; Krupka and Vener 1985; Metha *et al.* 1989). In advertisements for tranquillisers, the trend seems to be opposite to what it was in the 1970s: pictures of men seem to dominate (Thompson 1979; Krupka and Vener 1985). The trends in drug advertising and their implications for women will be further discussed in Chapter 5.

At the level of the *health care system* the interests of women have, in the words of Alford (1975), been pursued by 'public health advocates'. As indicated in Chapter 2, public health concerns tend to reinforce the absent presence of women rather than raise their use of psychotropics as a gendered issue.

In this chapter, we have attempted to offer a comprehensive theoretical framework on psychotropic drug use. This framework not only makes women users visible but also highlights the gendered character of this type of drug use. The remaining chapters will attempt to build upon this framework.

Chapter 5

Advertising as a representation of gendered moods

INTRODUCTION

Advertising constitutes one of the major mechanisms whereby producers of commodities in market-based societies reach potential consumers and create a market for their products. Advertising is, however, not merely a question of strict product information but, perhaps more importantly, a way in which commodities are transformed into signifiers of something which is highly valued in society or by the target group in question (Williams 1993). The purpose of this chapter is to uncover the discourses used in advertisements for psychotropic drugs. We will explore how drug advertisements construct the user and, thereby, constitute cultural representations of the user. Our discussion will begin with a review of advertisements as representations and we will then look at the portrayal of gender, gender roles and gender relationships in drug advertisements and to whom they are directed. Finally, we will present the findings from a study of gender portrayals in advertisements for psychotropic drugs in the major medical journals in the Nordic countries during the period 1975–93.

ADVERTISEMENTS AS CULTURAL REPRESENTATIONS

The body and its normal as well as pathological states and expressions are interpreted by the medical profession through the framework of biomedicine. The biomedical knowledge of the body is conveyed to this respective profession first through medical textbooks during professional socialisation and later through medical handbooks, and to the innovators within the profession itself through articles in medical journals. These medical texts not only portray the 'natural' body but also convey concealed notions about gender. These texts can be seen to be active and as constituents of social, indeed gendered relations (Smith 1990). The social construction of the body implies an agency, linking the 'natural' body and the cultural body (Shilling 1993:10). The medical profession is the major agency which constructs the human body by means of the 'medical gaze'. This implies a way of making the deep recesses of the body visible (Armstrong 1983, 1990). For many feminists, the construction of the body is tacitly a masculine endeavour and a way in which the female body is captured by the paradox of gender (Bordo 1993; Butler 1993). As feminist scholars have amply documented (e.g. Martin 1988, 1991), portrayals of the female body, especially the reproductive organs, tend to contain also broader values and stereotypical assumptions about women's position in society rather than merely neutral observations of the workings of bodily organs.

Advertising uses two ways to promote products: gender typing and metaphors. *Gender typing* of commodities has been a powerful strategy in selling products. For example, automobiles or alcoholic beverages are sold as a sign of masculinity, and detergents and household items as a sign of housewifery. The gender identification of products has created gendered markets for most commodities in modern society. In their study of gender stereotyping of products, Iyer and Debevec (1986) found that products were perceived generally as either exclusively masculine or feminine, although men and women tended to view items as being more often than not related to their own gender. As gender roles in society are gradually changing, companies are beginning to explore the possibilities of dual gender positioning (i.e. using both male- and female-directed positions) in their marketing as a way of expanding or creating new markets (Bellizzi and Milner (1991:72). Advertising researchers depict the ambiguity of the current situation as follows: 'The changing role of women in society has created a challenging task for advertisers – how to portray women in advertisements' (Leigh *et al*. 1987:54) because 'advertisers are finding it difficult to predict whether ads featuring alluring female models will be perceived as "sexy" or "sexist"' (Ford and LaTour 1993:43). As one group of researchers sums up the views on female gender portrayals in advertising: 'The issue of how best to communicate to women is thus problematic' (Leigh *et al.* 1987:55).

Research on advertising shows a marked shift from traditional gender portrayals in advertising during the period 1950–80 to more gender-neutral advertisements and more male gender positions, specifically since the 1980s.

One of the first studies of advertisements in American popular magazines (in 1970) showed women as buyers of cosmetics and household products, whereas men were depicted as buyers of more expensive products such as automobiles (Courtney and Lockeretz 1971). Four themes concerning female stereotypes surfaced in the advertisements: women's place was depicted as in the home; women did not make important decisions; women were dependent on their husbands; and women were perceived by men as sexual objects. These themes have continued to dominate the female gender portrayals, as documented in studies of gender stereotyping in popular magazines from the 1950s to the early 1980s (Belkaoui and Belkaoui 1976; Sullivan and O'Connor 1988). Recent research on health and wellness products demonstrates that females are more likely than males to be placed in submissive or unnatural positions; sexually displayed; emphasised through dismemberment of female body parts or subjects of violent imagery (Rudman and Hagiwara 1992; Rudman and Verdi 1993). Although women still feature in a social context where they have passive roles (i.e. they are displayed as sex objects, as dependent on men, as not making important decisions, as housewives), the images of women are becoming more varied. Research on long-term trends in advertisements reveals some changes in gender role display and current consumer preferences for gender role portrayals. Sullivan and O'Connor's (1988) study of advertisements in 1958, 1970 and 1983 in American magazines shows an increase of male portrayals for most products, including drugs. While drugs were sold primarily in 1958 and

1970 by female portrayals, the male ones dominated in 1983 (Sullivan and O'Connor 1988:185).

Recent advertising research has examined the reactions of both men and women to traditional and non-traditional gender portrayals in advertisements. There are two consistent trends: first, men seem to be more conservative and consistently favour the traditional. Second, women as a group are more positive towards non-traditional gender portrayals. By means of an experimental design, creating a male explicit, a female explicit and a neutral gender position for an automobile repair service shop, Bellizzi and Milner (1991) showed that men reacted less positively than women to a female explicit gender position, but men and women reacted similarly to male explicit positions. Prakash (1992:49–50) showed that men preferred advertisements in which men socialised in large groups and participated in competitive activities as well as in situations displaying traditional sex-roles of male–female interaction. Women preferred portrayals of themselves socialising in large or small groups, working by themselves or in intimate settings with other females or males. In exploring women's reactions to various female role portrayals, Leigh *et al.* (1987) found that the most effective advertisement was one in which the role portrayal in the advertisement was congruent with a woman's role orientation. Nevertheless, 'traditional women' appear to be more tolerant than 'modern women' to various female role portrayals (see also Ford and LaTour 1993). As the authors conclude: 'A "safe" strategy for a company faced with a vaguely defined target audience, or an inability to selectively reach distinct target segments, may be to use more modern female role portrayals' (Leigh *et al.* 1987:60).

Recent studies have explored the portrayal of gender relations in advertisements (Belknap and Leonard II 1991; Klassen *et al.* 1993) and examined changes over time (from 1972 to 1989). Although traditional portrayals of women tend to dominate, these have been decreasing since the early 1980s, while 'equality portrayals' are increasing (Klassen *et al.* 1993:36–7). There was, however, no empirical support for the widely held belief in a rise of advertisements that portray men in 'reverse-sex' relations, i.e. subordinate to women.

Finally, gender typing has constituted a major discourse whereby commodities are sold and target groups defined. Since the early 1980s, female gender portrayals in advertisements contain, however, a broader variety of female roles while male gender portrayals appear to have undergone little change. Nevertheless, male gender portrayals appear more frequently in the 1980s and 1990s than during the decades before and they tend, in fact, at present to dominate most products.

In addition to gender typing, *metaphors* constitute another theme in advertising. Here the term metaphor is used to denote a way of understanding and experiencing one phenomenon in terms of another (Lakoff and Johnson 1980). Metaphors work as a way of linking the concrete with the more immanent: connecting something abstract with the concrete commodity. For example, a sentiment or an ideal is portrayed as being harboured in a commodity, such as when an advertisement for a diamond ring is sold as a token of a man's love for a woman, or oatmeal cookies are presented as signifying true motherhood. Leiss and his colleagues (1986:241) contend, in their overview of the character of advertising, that the 'metaphor is the very heart of the basic communicative form used in modern advertising.'

How do gender portrayals and metaphors in drug advertisements compare to advertisements for everyday commodities and services? Before we begin to answer this question, two comments have to be made about the specific character of drug advertising. The first comment is that advertisements for prescribed drugs appear in medical journals and are not read by the actual consumer of the drug but specifically by the prescribing physician. The physicians act as a gatekeeping mechanism in the legal acquisition of prescribed drugs. The purpose of drug advertising is, therefore, to influence the physician's prescribing habits. As expected, drug advertisements seem to reach their target – the physicians. Walton (1980) examined the impact of 354 ads including 186 drugs on a panel of 1000 physicians and found that, in 95 per cent of the cases, identification of an advertisement was associated with positive prescribing. In fact, advertisements for minor tranquillisers had the highest 'success rate': 60 per cent of

physicians who were aware of the minor tranquilliser advertisements also prescribed the drug. This was in comparison to
approximately a third to a half of the physicians (within the
same panel) who reported an awareness of and prescribing in
other drug categories (Walton 1980:45). A review of the major
factors influencing drug prescribing has shown that advertising plays a major role apart from professionally related
ones, e.g. specialisation and colleague networks (Hemminki
1975).

As drug companies continuously introduce new drugs on
the market, physicians become dependent on commercial
sources for information about new drugs. Hence, physicians'
decisions about drug therapy are more related to the role
played by advertising and retailers of drugs than to medical
knowledge of the appropriate regimen (see Krupka and Vener
1985; Lexchin 1987, 1989). Furthermore, research has shown
that commercial sources are more important for general practitioners when they prescribe a new drug than for specialists,
who receive this information from medical sources (Peay and
Peay 1988, 1990).

In the United States, advertising of prescription drugs
directly to consumers has been allowed since 1985, although
strict guidelines are required. Studies indicate that about a
third of those surveyed recall having seen an advertisement
for prescribed medications during a specific year and were
positive about such advertising (Everett 1991; Alperstein and
Peyrot 1993).

The second comment concerning the specific character of
drug advertising is that it is far from a homogeneous commodity. Prescribed drugs cover a variety of diseases and
ailments which tend to strike women and men differently. The
question often pondered in research on drug advertisements is
whether or not advertisements are reflections of 'reality', i.e.
the gender distribution of those suffering from the chronic
illness in question. The futility of such a question becomes
evident when the metaphors of drug advertisements are examined. Here, the psychological appeal to physicians'
prescribing habits by means of metaphors is more blatant. The
metaphors assist in attaching a certain symbolic meaning to

each drug, and thereby influence the physicians' prescribing habits.

Use of stereotypical gender role portrayals is a common feature in drug advertising. This was confirmed in a number of studies of drug advertisements appearing in Anglo-Saxon medical journals in the 1970s. For example, Mant and Darroch (1975) observed that the gender roles depicted were stereotypical for all drug groups: men were shown as working and women as minding the home or in glamorous poses.

Advertisements for tranquillisers have been shown to be more gender biased than advertisements for other categories of drugs. In the 1970s, women were the dominant users shown in the advertisements for tranquillisers, while advertisements for other drugs had either a more even gender distribution or contained more men (Mant and Darroch 1975; Prather and Fidell 1975). Furthermore, women portrayed in the advertisements for tranquillisers were shown in stereotypical roles, often as depressed housewives (Seidenberg 1971; Prather and Fidell 1975; Chapman 1979). Prather and Fidell (1975) found that advertisements tended to depict men's need for tranquillisers as related to anxiety in their occupational role or to physical problems, while women's need for tranquillisers was related to diffuse symptoms.

Since the end of the 1970s, a new trend in the proportion of gender portrayal in drug advertising has been documented. A study of advertising for a variety of products in American magazines showed that men appeared in drug advertisements more often than women in 1983, in contrast to earlier years: 1958 and 1970 (Sullivan and O'Connor 1988). In their study of the gender distribution in prescription drug advertisements, Krupka and Vener (1985) showed a trend towards more gender-neutral portrayals in 1972, 1977 and 1982 and a decrease in the use of female gender portrayals. The same finding was confirmed in a study on gender portrayals in advertisements for oral hypoglycemics between 1963 and 1986 (Mehta *et al.* 1989). Krupka and Vener (1985:194) found that the gender depicted in the advertisements for drugs which treat the central nervous system changed from 52 per cent being neutral, 27 per cent male and 21 per cent female in 1972 to 65 per cent, 24 per cent and 11 per cent respectively in 1982. The same trend could be documented in a sample of drug advertisements drawn from three leading American medical journals between 1987 and 1991 which showed an over-representation of male gender portrayals (Leppard *et al.* 1993). The latter study showed, however, a gender difference in the type of psychotropics advertised: women dominated the gender portrayals in advertisements for hypnotics-sedatives, whereas men dominated the tranquilliser drug advertisements focusing on men in the workplace (Leppard *et al.* 1993:835).

Despite the trend towards more gender-neutral portrayals, the explicit gender portrayals continue to be stereotypical: they reflect the social relations of gender. Hawkins and Aber (1988, 1993) found that the pictures in drug advertisements in American medical journals in 1986 showed men and women differently. Women are stressed; the causes of stress are family, housework and menial tasks. On the other hand, men are portrayed as being stressed by work. A majority (68 per cent) of the workers are men. When women appear as workers, they are secretaries and waitresses. Women are caricatured twice as often as men and are portrayed naked in nearly a 4:1 ratio *vis-à-vis* men (Hawkins and Aber 1993:237).

Leppard and her colleagues' (1993:834) study of drug advertisements in three leading American medical journals between 1987 and 1991 found that both males and females were portrayed stereotypically, but male representations were more frequently so than female ones. The authors' reflection on this finding is that women's roles in society have changed. More and different roles for women are shown, whereas the male work role is still the major gender portrayal for men.

Metaphors, here implying pictures without portrayal of humans, constitute a major communicative device in drug advertising. Studies of metaphors, appearing in drug advertisements, are generally analysed by means of a semiological approach to decode the symbols and tacit messages (Prather 1991; Leiss *et al.* 1986). For example, Chapman (1979) analysed the metaphors and myths in advertisements for psychotropics in a medical journal in Australia. He found that the advertisements propagated several myths: psychotropics are a natural part of the everyday life of the elderly and of housewives; the missing piece of a broken life; and a flight ticket from problems. These metaphors were illustrated by concrete pictures. Goldman and Montagne (1986) have shown that drug companies use abstract and visual metaphors in their advertisements for psychotropics. Drug advertisements attempt to associate certain mental states with visual symbols – for example, depression with a picture of a single eye.

Metaphors tend to structure people's experience and understanding of drugs and drug use. Montagne (1991, 1988) has presented a review of the metaphors used by scholars, health personnel and journalists to characterise tranquillisers and their use. He argues that the metaphors reflect cultural perceptions of anxiety and nervousness. Tranquillisers are, for example, perceived as magic bullets, a travel ticket to tranquillity and normality, or an instrument to repair broken machinery. Aside from these positive images, tranquillisers also have negative connotations – as enslavers or strait-jackets. Use of tranquillisers has also been conceptualised in both positive and negative terms as, for example, a chemical vacation, an artificial paradise, an evil necessity or a plague (Montagne 1991:54)

In his impressionistic review of advertisements for psychotropic drugs in 'major professional journals' during the period 1955–80, Neill (1989) puts forward an important viewpoint, interpreting the advertisements as having mainly a therapeutic function for the physician. He sees a shift, however, in the message of the early psychotropic drug advertisements to that of the later ones. Earlier drug advertisements indicated that the drugs enhanced the physician's (in this case, the psychiatrist's) own personality and therapeutic qualities. Later on the therapeutic function of the advertisements, Neill (1989:337) argues, was to reassure the psychiatrist that the drug rather than his or her professional role had the power to cure the patient.

In the light of the above discussion, the review of the literature on drug advertisements shows two themes and two concomitant methodological approaches. One theme is the gender typing of products, which has been documented by means of quantitative content analysis either longitudinally or cross-sectionally for several journals. The findings of this approach indicate that gender-neutral portrayals have become increasingly common, but that those which contain gender-explicit positions tend to portray stereotypical gender roles for both males and females. The other theme is the use of metaphors in drug advertising, documented by means of a qualitative approach. The purpose of the latter approach is to de-construct texts and images in order to uncover the tacit meaning or discourse.

In the following discussions, we will apply these two approaches and themes to illustrate how the patient's need for a psychotropic medication is constructed by the pharmaceutical companies in advertisements which appeared in the major medical journals in the Nordic countries during the past two decades.

ARE SCANDINAVIAN MOODS GENDERED? REPRESENTATIONS IN PSYCHOTROPIC DRUG ADVERTISING

A sociological inquiry into the nature of psychotropic drug advertising in the Nordic countries (i.e. Denmark, Finland, Norway and Sweden) is of interest for at least two major reasons. The first is that research on psychotropic drug advertising has been limited mainly to Anglo-Saxon medical journals. In this kind of research, the notion of women's sphere as the home and men's as the workplace has characterised the investigations, while women's recent entry into the labour market has raised a number of questions concerning their future role and health. The Nordic countries have not experienced as vivid a cultural norm of the institution of housewifery. In comparison to women in an Anglo-Saxon context, Nordic and specifically Finnish women's entry into the labour market came relatively early in this century (Pohls 1990; Rantalaiho 1993) and was followed by family-policy programmes to support women's dual role. In this respect, the Nordic countries offer an opportunity to see whether the portrayal of modern female and male gender roles has permeated drug advertising. It is also to be expected that the high proportion of women physicians in these countries, ranging from 26 per cent in Norway to 46 per cent in Finland in 1994, will have an influence on these portrayals. The advertisements are directed after all at the physician, not the patient. Not only the gender portrayal of the user but also the gender portrayal of the provider is, therefore, important.

The second reason for an interest in psychotropic drug advertising in Nordic medical journals is that all Nordic countries have similar health care systems, based on the so-called Nordic model. The population is covered by a universal and comprehensive sickness insurance, and the public sector dominates health care delivery. The majority of physicians practise in the public sector as salaried employees. Furthermore, the costs of prescribed drugs are reimbursed partially or totally by insurance schemes. Hence, neither shortcomings in access nor in the financing of health services have a major influence over the use of health care or drugs.

The data on advertisements for psychotropic drugs derive from two separate studies of psychotropic drug advertisements appearing in the major medical journals in the Nordic countries between 1975 and 1993. The results covering the period from 1975 to 1985 will be used as a basis for a discussion of the portrayal of gender roles in psychotropic advertisements in the same journals in 1993.

Psychotropic drug advertising the Scandinavian way, 1975–85

The first study was a quantitative content analysis of all the advertisements for psychotropic drugs which appeared in the Finnish (*Suomen lääkärilehti*, N = 327), Swedish (*Läkartidningen*, N = 1009) and Danish (*Ugeskrift for læger*, N = 2059) major medical journals between 1975 and 1985. The Danish journal contained the most advertisements per issue (3.5), followed by the Swedish (1.9) and the Finnish ones (0.8). Only the Finnish, Swedish and Danish journals were chosen in this study because previous studies have shown that these three countries have the most marked differences in sales and self-reported use of psychotropics. Norway was excluded from the analysis because its sales statistics and prevalence figures of drug use resemble those of Sweden. The same scheme was used for classifying the advertisements in the three national medical journals. Three major themes were used in the classification of these advertisements: 'metaphors', 'patients' and 'other'. In this context, *metaphors* are pictures or drawings which portray something other than the concrete medication or the user of the drug. Metaphors carry a symbolic meaning by depicting, for example, insects, birds, landscape and parts of houses (e.g. an open door, a dilapidated house, etc.). The category *patient* portrays a person who either experiences the symptoms which the medication alleviates or the effects of the medication. The category *other* contains advertisements which show only textual information, a drug bottle or a diagram of the effects of the drug, but which do not contain pictures with symbolic meaning or with patients or providers. In the following review *only* the major results will be highlighted, as a full report of the results of this study (Riska and Hägglund 1991; Hägglund 1991) and a separate analysis of the advertisements for minor tranquillisers in the Nordic countries between 1975 and 1985 (Hägglund and Riska 1993) have been presented already elsewhere.

The relative distribution of advertisements for different psychotropic drug groups varied widely between the Nordic countries, apart from antidepressants which constituted about 20 per cent of the advertisements. As Table 5.1 shows, 40 per cent of the advertisements in the Finnish journal were for neuroleptics, a strong antipsychotic drug, while both the drugs composing the so-called minor tranquillisers based on the benzodiazepine compounds (i.e. tranquillisers and hypnotics-sedatives) composed together an equally large proportion. The minor tranquillisers constituted around 65 per cent of the psychotropic advertisements in the Swedish and the Danish journals.

About half the pictures in the advertisements for psycho-tropic drugs in the Danish and the Finnish medical journals contained a metaphor, compared to a third in the Swedish journal. The themes which appeared in the metaphors followed no systematic pattern by drug group. The most frequent portrayals were: nature, animals, birds, insects, vehicles, technology, window, door, puzzle, watch, science fiction, art books, demons, broken pieces and night pictures. The themes

Table 5.1 Distribution (%) of advertisements for psychotropics by drug category and major themes in the main Danish, Finnish and Swedish medical journals, 1975–85

Content of advertisement	Denmark	Finland	Sweden
Drug category			
Neuroleptics	16	40	18
Antidepressants	17	20	17
Tranquillisers	29	19	34
Hypnotics-sedatives	37	21	31
Several of the above	1	–	–
Major themes			
Metaphor	51	51	33
Patient	17	27	22
Other	32	22	45
Total (%)	100	100	100
N	2059	327	1009

indicated either the reasons for the illness (demons, broken pieces of a life, sleepless nights) or the effects of the drug (a door, a window or a ship offering the possibility of a new life).

In the category 'other' the Swedish journal had a comparatively high proportion (30 per cent) of advertisements depicting the package of the drug, as compared to the other journals. Such advertisements come as close as possible to factual information about a drug. By contrast, the theme of a metaphor and a patient are interpreted as signifiers of the social construction of the user of the drug. A *patient* was portrayed in around one-fifth to one-fourth of the advertisements for psychotropic drugs. Women constituted approximately half the patients depicted in the advertisements for all journals (see Table 5.2). The portrayal of gender varied by drug group in the three journals. For example, 63 per cent of the men were depicted in advertisements for neuroleptics in the Finnish journal, compared to only 10 per cent of the women (not shown in Table 5.1). By contrast, women were featured most frequently in advertisements for hypnotics-sedatives (42 per cent of the women) in the Finnish journal. The latter pattern was also found in the Danish journal, where half the female gender portrayals were for hypnotics-sedatives whereas men (43 per cent) were clustered in advertisements for tranquillisers. The Swedish journal showed the most even distribution of female and male gender portrayals between the four drug groups (Hägglund 1991:163).

About 80 per cent of the depicted patients were middle-aged in the Finnish and Danish material, but slightly less than half the patients were in this age group in the Swedish material (Table 5.2). Instead, one-fourth of the patients in the Swedish material were elderly, a category with

Table 5.2 Distribution (%) of pictures of patients by gender, age and job status in the advertisements for psychotropics appearing in the Danish, Finnish and Swedish medical journals, 1975–85

Characteristics/Gender	Denmark	Finland	Sweden
Women only	50	55	47
Men only	49	31	41
Both men and women	1	14	12
Age			
Child	2	–	–
Youth	2	–	3
Middle-aged	80	81	46
Elderly	5	14	28
Several age groups	–	5	6
Unknown	11	–	17
Job status			
Working	11	30	15
Non-working	49	23	70
Outside of a social context	40	45	13
Other	–	2	2
Total (%)	100	100	100
N	349	87	217

a much lower visibility in the Finnish (14 per cent) and the Danish (5 per cent) material. Closer examination of the data revealed that elderly people appeared in advertisements for neuroleptics in the Danish and the Finnish material. In the Swedish journal, over half the elderly were women, a third were men and the remainder depicted elderly couples. By contrast, elderly women did not appear at all as a leading theme in the Finnish material. Instead, more than half the advertisements depicting elderly people showed an elderly couple and the remainder showed elderly men. In the Danish material 74 per cent of the pictures of the elderly showed a woman, 10 per cent depicted a man and the remainder a couple.

At the other end of the age spectrum were children and the young, who were not portrayed in the Finnish material at all. Some pictures of young people (approximately 15–22 years old) appeared in the Swedish and the Danish journals: they were all boys in the Danish journal, in advertisements for antidepressants; there were both boys and girls in the Swedish journal and they appeared in advertisements for neuroleptics, hypnotics-sedatives and antidepressants.

The Danish journal was the only one that carried advertisements depicting a small child as the consumer of psychotropic drugs. The picture showed a girl about four years old, who was crying and the text indicated that the marketed tranquilliser 'alleviated cramp'.

The working status of the patients portrayed in the advertisements showed that the Swedish journal had the highest proportion of patients (70 per cent) who were not working, i.e. the picture showed either an in- or outdoor leisure activity, or a more general setting which was not a place of work. About two-fifths of the patients in the Finnish and the Danish journals were depicted without a social context. The largest proportion of patients shown at a workplace appeared in the Finnish material (see Table 5.2). These advertisements were also recent: the first advertisements with a working person appeared in the journal in 1983. Each person shown at a workplace was a woman in the Finnish journal. Seventy-three per cent of these working women were shown in a teaching role and the remainder in office work. All the pictures of women in a teaching role were in advertisements for hypnotics-sedatives, while all the office workers were shown in advertisements for tranquillisers. By contrast, no man was shown in a workplace context in the Finnish journal. In fact, 85 per cent of the patients shown not working were men. Men were depicted as suffering from severe mental health problems which were not illustrated as generated or alleviated by a special social context. The gender differences in the social context of the patient were, however, related to the type of psychotropic advertised for each gender. As shown above, most male patients in the Finnish journal appeared in advertisements for neuroleptics, which in general are prescribed for symptoms of severe psychiatric illness. By contrast, 63 per cent of the women appeared in advertisements for tranquillisers and hypnotics-sedatives which are used to alleviate anxiety and insomnia.

In the Danish journal, all those depicted in a workplace setting were either teaching or doing office work. The majority of the women were shown in a teaching role (83 per cent). They appeared in advertisements for hypnotics-sedatives. The remainder were depicted doing office work in advertisements which marketed tranquillisers.

In the Swedish journal, men were shown as office workers mainly in advertisements for tranquillisers and neuroleptics. Women were doing office work and teaching; they all appeared in advertisements for tranquillisers. Only the Swedish journal assigned women to the role of housewife and these all appeared in 1975.

The representation of the users of psychotropics in the Nordic countries in the 1990s

In order to compare advertisements for psychotropics in the major medical journals in the Nordic countries in the 1970s and 1980s with the 1990s, all the advertisements for psychotropics in the 1993 issues of the Finnish (*Suomen lääkärilehti*, N = 57), Swedish (*Läkartidningen*, N = 62), Danish (*Ugeskrift for læger*, N = 122) and Norwegian (*Tidsskrift for den norske laegeforening*, N = 55) major medical journals were examined. We chose to include the Norwegian journal in this later study because we wanted a more comprehensive picture of the current situation. The largest number of advertisements for psychotropics per issue appeared again in the Danish journal (2.4), followed by the Norwegian (1.8), Finnish (1.6) and Swedish (1.2) journals. The Danish journal also featured the greatest variety of advertisements (N = 29) as compared to the Finnish (N = 16), Norwegian (N = 10) and Swedish (N = 10) journals.[1]

Table 5.3 shows the distribution of the three themes in the four medical journals. Metaphors dominate advertisements for psychotropics in the Finnish medical journal during both periods (51 per cent and 65 per cent respectively) (see Tables 5.1 and 5.3). The Danish journal shows a slight decline in the use of metaphors in advertisements. From previously making up half the advertisements in earlier years, they constituted one-third in 1993. The latter proportion is also found in the distribution of themes in the Swedish journal, but the level of

Table 5.3 Distribution (%) of pictures by major themes and pictures of patients by gender in advertisements for psychotropics in the Nordic major medical journals in 1993

Content	Denmark	Finland	Norway	Sweden
Major theme				
Metaphor	36	65	–	37
Patient	48	32	100	52
Other	16	3	–	11
Total (%)	100	100	100	100
N	122	57	55	62
Gender of the patient				
Women only	53	100	78	94
Men only	8	–	5	6
Both women and men	31	–	17	–
Unknown	8	–	–	–
Total (%)	100	100	100	100
N	59	18	55	32

advertisements containing a metaphor has remained relatively constant over the years (33 per cent and 37 per cent). Metaphors were not used at all in advertisements for psychotropics in the Norwegian journal in 1993.

The portrayal of patients in advertisements for psychotropics constitutes approximately one-third of the advertisements in the Finnish journal between 1975 and 1993. The use of patients in advertising for psychotropics rose, however, from approximately one-fifth to one-half of the advertisements in the Swedish and the Danish journals. One reason for the marked increase in the portrayal of patients in the latter two journals is the declining use of factual features, i.e. the category 'other'. In the Norwegian journal, *all* advertisements for psychotropics portrayed a patient in 1993.

In this context, two questions arise: Who is the assumed user in 1993? Are there any major variations in the representations between the journals? In all four journals women dominate the representation of the user. The Finnish, Swedish and Norwegian portrayals convey a rather homogeneous notion of the female user, while the Danish journal contains a broader range of social types. For example, *all* users in the Finnish journal are women (see Table 5.3), most about 45 years old. In nearly all the advertisements, the women are active, providing evidence of the beneficial effect of the drug. One advertisement for a hypnotic shows an alert and content female teacher who has obviously had a good night's sleep. A few passive women were used to advertise a tranquilliser, which the text indicates is for feelings of panic. In general, the women in the Finnish advertisements appear to be middle-class or professional, unrepresentative of the female population at large.

Almost all the users in the Swedish journal (94 per cent) are women but they are portrayed as passive – or with only their heads revealed (see Table 5.3). They are around 50 years old, well-kempt in terms of make-up, hair-style and clothing, and they give the impression of belonging to the upper middle class. There is one advertisement for an antidepressant featuring a middle-class male of about 50. He is sitting at a table with a somewhat gloomy expression and he seems to be contemplating a model of a sailing ship. The general impression of the users in the Swedish journal, regardless of gender, is that they are passive, either because they are experiencing the effects of the drug or because they need it.

On the surface, the Danish journal shows a much broader variety of gender roles and gender relations (see Table 5.3). Approximately half the advertisements portray women only and they are active; for example, cycling, shopping, working, walking, reading, about to drive a car. They are not as well groomed as, for example, the Finnish and Swedish women. Their hair falls naturally, they wear no make-up and their clothing is typically lower middle class. (There is one exception – an upper middle-class woman who is depicted as getting ready to drive her car.)

The users in the Danish journal are portrayed as individuals who are (noticeably more often than in the other journals) engaged in an interaction with another person. While the other journals portray the user in a non-social context, the Danish portrayals indicate that the medication enables the user to fulfil his or her obligations to primary group relations. This is depicted in a typical Danish context: one advertisement for an antidepressant shows a 40ish middle-class male giving his four-year-old daughter a ride on a bike in an urban context (most probably to her day-care centre). The innuendo here is unclear: is this an 'equality ad' (i.e. he is, with the assistance of the drug, able to fulfil demands for gender equality) or is this an example of 'role reversal' (i.e. he can perform the traditional female role)?

The text of the advertisement with the cycling male is typical of the genre in Danish advertisements. The text says: 'Long-term treatment for depression' and continues 'Stable effect: a reoccurrence can, for the individual depressive patient, have *catastrophic social consequences* in terms of unemployment, marriage breakdown and suicide. At the same time, depressive episodes are related to massive *economic costs* for society.' What is typical of the Danish texts is that they are lengthy and generally involve a social theme, while the language in the other journals is laconic, e.g. 'Out of depression' being a common theme (the Finnish version is somewhat crude and reads in translation 'Knock out the blues', i.e. *Turpiin depikselle*).

Along with the Norwegian journal, the Danish journal portrays gender relationships, i.e. showing men and women together. However, for the Danish journal this portrayal constitutes 31 per cent. In half the pictures women and men are shown in situations where they are interacting, and it is even unclear who is the user. The other half depict a man as the saviour of the depressed woman. There are three versions of this advertisement portraying the gender relationship: the man, the hero Harlequin, assists the depressed heroine Columbine to perform her traditional female role again.[2] It is unclear, however, whether Harlequin symbolises the drug, the physician or the male player, with whom the woman is supposed to act out her 'normal' female role. What is clear, however, is the female gender of the user. When these implicit female user portrayals are added to the portrayals of explicit female users, women constitute 73 per cent of the depicted users of psychotropics in Danish advertisements.

The Norwegian journal differs from the other three in that the advertisements feature only patients. For example, metaphors do not appear at all. The majority of the users are women but a range of female roles is covered: a retired woman, a mother with her baby son, passive and active women, mostly around 40 years old. Their appearance also varies, from the worn-out attitudes of some severely depressed women, a cosy farmer's wife, to an urban, well-dressed, female secretary in expensive clothes and heavy make-up. The latter is featured in two advertisements and one reads: 'She could not do her job: not because she was depressed but because of the side effects'; the other says that the drug 'does not lower the psychomotor capacities one is dependent on at work', alluding to her use of a personal computer. The same company features an advertisement with a man driving a car and simultaneously handling a mobile telephone. Here we are not informed that by taking the drug he can perform his job, but that the drug 'does not lower the psychomotor capacities one is dependent on in *everyday life*' (our italics).

In the advertisements for hypnotics one can spot the effects of the public debate on the dependency-producing effects of benzodiazepines. This issue is addressed differently in the four journals: some allude to it in euphemistic terms, others confront it explicitly. For example, the Finnish advertisements only touch on the issue by calling the drug 'safe' without using the word dependency at all. One advertisement reads: 'Proven safe when used correctly. Good nights and good mornings.' The Swedish advertisement reads: 'Balance with [drug X]: without drug dependency and withdrawal effects . . . New strategies, new expectations'; and another reads 'Good nights without dependency'. The Danish advertisements also mention explicitly 'no dependency effect', 'rebound effect', 'tolerance level', 'dependency', 'side effects'. One of the most straightforward statements appears, in fact, in a Danish advertisement for a drug based on diazepam. It reads: 'Does the prescribing of [drug X] require nerves of steel?', alluding here to the doctor's choice of regimen. The text continues further down the page: 'Benzodiazepines are often maligned medications for ameliorating anxiety. But if the doctor and the patient have a clear agreement concerning the duration and intensity of treatment, there are seldom any side effects . . . If anxiety is to be treated with benzodiazepines, do it with a clear conscience.'

The above examples of the texts where hypnotics are advertised show that the pharmaceutical companies have incorporated the criticisms of benzodiazepines in the advertising context. In fact, the medical and social discourses, identified in the criticism of the 1980s (see Chapter 2), have been capitalised on and used as a major advertising strategy. By co-opting and capitalising on the medical and public criticism of benzodiazepines into drug advertising, the pharmaceutical companies have not only neutralised criticism but also, more importantly, redefined it into a phenomenon which the drug industry appears to have addressed and solved. The drugs are thus marketed by means of this redefinition.

GENDERING TEXTS AND GENDERING POTENTIAL USE

Illustrations of the potential user and gender typing of the user constitute a major advertising strategy, whereby pharmaceutical companies prepare a market for psychotropics in the Nordic countries. Leaving aside the Finnish journal, portrayal of the user of the medication has become more frequent compared to the more factual information provided in the 1970s and 1980s. In the words of Goffman (1976; see also Belknap and Leonard 1991; Klassen *et al.* 1993), the advertisements are gendered and the 'gender display' refers to conventional portrayals of the culturally established attributes of sex. Our examination of gender and gender roles displayed in psychotropic drug advertising in the Nordic medical journals shows that female gender positions dominate. Drug advertising constructs gendered moods and enhances the creation of a female-dependent product. This is particularly evident in the Finnish journal which showed only female users, although the prevalence of the use of psychotropics in the population indicates almost no gender difference.

What, then, can be said of the gender roles depicted, if we use the three categories – traditional, reverse-sex and equality ads – used by Klassen *et al.* (1993) in their study of gender roles and gender relations in advertisements? The modern roles clearly characterise female users. In the Nordic context this means the portrayal of an active, middle-class woman who with the assistance of the drug is capable of maintaining her independence as a woman without venturing into the male domain. As a consequence, the 'reverse-sex ad' appeared only with a male, and only one advertisement of working life featured an 'equality ad'. Both the 'reverse-sex ad' and the 'equality ad' featured in the Danish journal, and such advertisements did not appear at all in the other three.

The overall impression of gender portrayal in drug advertising in the Nordic countries is that stereotypical female gender portrayals appear today more in hormone replacement advertisements than in those for psychotropics. The 'iconic expression' (Goffman 1976) hidden in our gender portrayals is that Nordic women are governed as much by their 'nerves', or uncomfortable moods, as by their hormones. Nevertheless, both the mood and the hormone discourses reflect a viewpoint called 'biological materialism' which is used to explain female gender behaviour. The 'mood discourse' constructs the reason for women's mental instability as being concealed within women's 'nerves' indicating the 'invisible femininity' of the nervous system (see Theriot 1993:10). In our review of the literature on women's use of psychotropics in Chapter 3, this discourse was called, in that context, the 'women-are-expressive hypothesis'. In comparison, the 'hormone discourse' reinforces the biological notion of the female gender, a perspective called 'gynaecological essentialism' (Theriot 1993:12). The latter type of essentialism ties women's gender and mental health to their reproductive organs. Both the mood and the hormone discourses confirm the notion of the innate nature of women's behaviour and health. Nevertheless, drug advertising is part of the cultural process whereby the body is assigned its gender attributes, which the medical discourse legitimates and confirms.

Our Nordic study of advertising for psychotropics showed that, compared with the results of a previous study (Riska and Hägglund 1991), there is a gradual shift in advertising from tranquillising women to showing the need for treating depressed women. Women presenting with signs of depression are likely to be prescribed the new antidepressants such as Prozac (based on fluoxetine hydrochloride) introduced on the US market in 1987 – the new wonder drug of the 1990s (Concar 1994). It is believed that Prozac not only restores depressed people to their 'premorbid self' but also transforms them into feeling 'better than well'. An American psychiatrist, Peter Kramer (1993:15), has coined the term 'cosmetic psychopharmacology' to indicate the therapeutic potential of psychotropic drugs like Prozac. Kramer suggests that the popularity of antidepressants like Prozac lies in the change of social norms in society:

> because we value the assertive woman and shake our heads over the long-suffering self-sacrificer. Perhaps medication now risks playing a role that psychotherapy was accused of playing in the past: it allows a person to achieve happiness through conformity to contemporary norms.
>
> (Kramer 1993:40)

The ethical implications of such a use of drugs are serious and should be considered more publicly if their use is going to replicate the trends in the use of the benzodiazepines, the wonder drug of the 1960s.

In the following chapter, we turn our attention to a discussion of the social construction of psychotropic drug use from the viewpoint of the individual as an analytical site. In that context, we provide a comprehensive picture of psychotropic drug users, some who have used 'this wonder drug of the 1960s'.

NOTES

1   In Denmark, the advertisements fell into the following groups: 37 per cent antidepressants, 42 per cent tranquillisers and 21 per cent hypnotics. In Finland, 39 per cent antidepressants, 28 per cent tranquillisers and 33 per cent hypnotics. In Sweden, 28 per cent antidepressants, 32 per cent tranquillisers, 29 per cent hypnotics and 11 per cent neuroleptics. In Norway, all the advertisements were for antidepressants.

2   The two characters belong to an institution in Danish culture: the pantomime theatre, established in 1874 at Tivoli, an amusement park in the centre of Copenhagen. This outdoor theatre carries on the legacy of *commedia dell'arte* and shows a much loved, ritual play each day at Tivoli. Any Dane would thus be able to grasp the connotation of the advertisement.

Chapter 6

Analysing long-term use
Users' narratives

INTRODUCTION

In this chapter we turn our attention to users and examine their personal accounts of psychotropic drug use. These accounts illustrate the 'individual layer of analysis' in the social construction of psychotropic drug use, as detailed in our theoretical framework in Chapter 4. The overall aim of this chapter is to provide a picture of psychotropic drug users, in which their beliefs about, attitudes towards and perceptions of psychotropic drug use become visible. The first part of the chapter focuses on issues related to becoming a long-term user. We will develop concepts such as the *discursive subject* and the *narrative*. Here, along with Conrad (1990), we believe that there is a need to spell out more specifically an insider's perspective on suffering and ill health. With special reference to the gendering of psychotropic drug use, we aim to break what Zola (1991:2) calls the 'structured silence of personal bodily experience'. The second half of the chapter looks at our empirical study.

The personal narratives of our respondents reflect the lives of those involved in long-term drug use. In this context, we look at some of the health reasons as well as life events related to our respondents' drug use. Within the structure of the narrative, we aim to highlight the importance of analyses of users which problematise gender.

BECOMING A LONG-TERM USER OF PSYCHOTROPICS

The widespread use of benzodiazepines, as new forms of psychotropic drugs, was established through a privileging process. On pharmacological grounds, they were valued over barbiturates because they had been perceived as less dangerous in terms of both overdose and addiction potential. As the new 'medicines for the mind' (Curran and Golombok 1985), they were appreciated by patients and doctors alike as a successful way of dealing with all sorts of physical as well as psychological ills. Gradually, a mystique developed and surrounded the use of minor tranquillisers: they were 'idealised' for what they could do for both the users and the providers (Medawar 1992).

For users, tranquillisers became a restorative – the nearest thing to bottled happiness (Melville 1984). Patients experienced a calming effect on their feelings of anxiety and tension. Media and popular representations of these drugs promoted the idea that one's everyday misfortunes would benefit from this type of medical attention (Prather 1991:122).

While the 'real business of medicine tends to be limited to physical pain, microbes, tissue pathology, viruses' (Blum et al. 1981:17), the notion that physicians, by dispensing these psychoactive drugs, could provide a 'cure' for emotional pain developed. Theoretically, physicians are not only trained but are also supposed to cure. These drugs became a visible sign of the physician's power to cure. Regardless of this fact, what was, in reality, being 'cured' or 'medicated' had more to do with patients' lack of adherence to social norms than any biological pathology. Nevertheless, physicians appeared as more understanding, humane, resourceful and concerned, as these drugs became a symbol of the power of modern medical technology in a pure and potent form (Montagne 1988, 1991).

This mystique was broken when the users and the public received messages that minor tranquillisers were no longer the 'once safe alternative to barbs' but had adverse effects as well as dependency potential (Hamlin and Hammersley 1989a, 1989b; Gudex 1991). But that health damage (from drugs), viewed either as dependency from the physician's point of view or addiction from the patient's (Drummond 1991), remained a hidden issue for a number of years should not be surprising. Prescription drug users, particularly compliant ones, tend to emphasise the positive rather than the negative effects (e.g. addictive potential) of their medicines (Herxheimer and Stimson 1981). Moreover, the medicinal use of minor tranquillisers created, soon after their introduction on the market, a type of 'benzodiazepine bonanza' (Tyrer 1974) within the medical profession.

In this context, we argue that becoming a long-term user entails a complex social process. It can be viewed within the context of changes in prescribing practices, the social acceptability of psychoactive drugs and the social norms surrounding the behaviour of gendered subjects. On a deeper dimension, this process highlights an (at times) enigmatic, social matrix in which these gendered subjects (e.g. psychotropic drug users) are positioned in social spaces in which they ask themselves or are asked by others, 'What is wrong?'

THE NEED FOR 'RESTORING THE SUBJECT'

In pursuit of the 'subject', Plummer (1983:5) wants sociology to pay tribute to human subjectivity and creativity – 'showing how individuals respond to social constraints and actively assemble their social worlds'. He argues that there have been movements in sociology to remove the subject from discourse by making 'it' a pre-defined entity with specific social or psychological properties. Thus, an important approach to understanding human life (i.e. a clear focus on the subject) has been persistently minimised, maligned and rendered marginal. Plummer argues that while our postmodernist culture is discovering a broader, more available, cultured individuality, we need a methodology which reflects this new emergence of individuality and which takes subjectivity and the lived life as its cornerstone.

In a similar vein of thinking but through the lens of medical sociology, Figlio (1987:77) argues that 'medical sociology needs to recover its lost subject'. Focusing on this lost subject, Silverman (1987:135) notes the importance of seeing the individual as a 'constituted subject' – that is, 'a subject constituted in the specific institutional and discursive practices of medicine'. Silverman's proposal echoes Turner's (1987:212) stated overall need for sociological analyses to work at three designated levels – that of the individual's experiences, social values and institutions, and the macrosocietal – in order to gain a full understanding of any health issue.

What the above perspectives do is to ensure that the 'subject' being spoken about in either general or medical sociology has the possibility of retaining, what we call, *discursive subjectivity*. Here, discursive subjectivity refers to how rational human beings evaluate their personal sense of routine and order in the social surroundings in which they find themselves. Discursive subjectivity is all about the ways that human beings are marked by analytical reasoning as individuals, as members of various social groups and by society. But, for long-term psychotropic drug users, discursive subjectivity is rooted in what Armstrong (1990:1227) calls 'the discourse of suffering'.

Here it should be noted that discursive subjectivity differs dramatically from what we earlier identified as 'voluntarism' in our discussion on user-oriented perspectives in Chapter 3. While both concepts, voluntarism and discursive subjectivity, focus on user rationality, they are based on different assumptions. On the one hand, voluntarism assumes that discourse formation is primarily an individualistic endeavour (i.e. going on in the mind of the subject). A subject's rationality appears within a social vacuum in which there is no space to see how society imposes various limitations on many individuals' (i.e. women, people of colour, mentally ill people) use of rationality and ultimately 'free choice'. On the other hand, discursive subjectivity implies that individuals with rationality, as well as varying limitations on exercising their rationality, speak as 'fettered' subjects bound within a variety of discourses or different fields of power/knowledge. But, most important, to speak as a subject means not only that the experiencing individual needs to speak, but also that this speaking is a social endeavour involving others.

Our task is, therefore, to ensure that the users observed in the field of psychotropic drugs retain discursive subjectivity. We aim to strengthen their status as subjects, a status challenged by the imposition of a deviant label which has given users, particularly women users, little room to speak as real experiencing persons. We attempt, therefore, to create a view of psychotropic drug use from the perspective of users themselves. Our way of doing this is to apply a concept, narrative, in order to analyse their social lives and, at times, personal troubles.

THE CONCEPT OF NARRATIVE

Linked with the notion of the subject, the concept of *narrative* is a fruitful one in analysing an 'insider's perspective' on health behaviour (Conrad 1990), specifically psychotropic drug use. Robinson's (1990) work defines the personal narrative as 'the process of subjectively placing the nature of illness in the temporal context of an individual's life'. Robinson roots his thinking in 'grounded theory', a case study approach, based on the earlier classical work of Glaser and Strauss (1967). This standpoint involves the extrapolation of patterned perceptions, elicited from a collection of a similar set of cases, while this approach can also be used to address how chronicity affects people's self-concepts within their illness experiences (Charmaz 1990).

In this context, the narrative can be used with special reference to long-term psychotropic users for two related theoretical reasons. First, it helps to make links between the subjective experience of illness and the fabrication of identity in this particular field of interest. Second, it helps to illuminate gendered concerns, concerns we want to emphasise when looking at psychotropic drug use.

Narrative creation and the fabrication of identity: the thinking and acting subject

There is a trend in sociology which emphasises a concern for individual lives and a 'new' pluralism, the latter extending 'the boundaries of what is acceptable, even if normality remains rigidly fixed as ever' (Evans 1993:6). In this light, subjective chronicling makes possible the construction of a narrative of self that is in line with the increasingly democratised and reordered sphere of one's personal life (Giddens 1991). Implicitly, the subjects and the codes in narrative construction have shifted (Evans 1993). This means that the use of the personal narrative allows one to speak about the past experiences of ordinary people who are not white, male, heterosexual, etc. or members of legitimised social groups, but who themselves are active participants in popular culture. This type of study embodies the social and reaffirms the centrality of certain general themes in the lives of individuals (Rosenau 1992).

Here, questions concerning the origins of the 'subject' located within the context of a variety of discriminating discourses arise. In this context, Armstrong (1993) demonstrates that the fabrication of identities through different public health regimes has circumscribed spaces for physical bodies and the psychosocial, allowing the emergence of individual differences as well as 'thinking and acting subjects'. This means that narratives of health and illness emerge from the space of surveillance which privileges society's need for healthy bodies and delineates the psychosocial space of interpersonal hygiene – a space which extends the notion of health promotion to all, regardless of health status.

Long-term psychotropic drug users may benefit from the new political appreciation of healthy bodies and increased knowledge of the dangers of prescription drugs as well as become more critical of their own drug use. Others may sense the need for increased levels of social and psychological competence in the management of everyday life and take psychotropics to maintain healthy bodies. This need appears consistent with what has been identified as a cultural stereotype of the professional middle class needing to be in control and in good physical and psychological health (Crawford 1984). Nevertheless, long-term psychotropic drug users embody a type of lifestyle which becomes visible in society as one demanding increased surveillance. The boundaries between drug-using (both legal and illegal) and non drug-using members of society are delineated by surveillance measures, based on cautionary idioms (i.e. 'Just say "no"!') and social norms of drug use (i.e. 'Drug use is dangerous.'). Hence, drug users are thrust into the space of surveillance which generates an awareness of drug-use 'traffic' for concerned social authorities (Dorn and Murji 1991) and, specifically, in which drug users appear as 'bad' thinking and 'anti-social' acting subjects.

In this context, we contend that the use of personal narratives can be valuable in allowing psychotropic drug users to speak as thinking and acting subjects – as ordinary, rational beings rather than as deviant or marginalised people. Thus, their *narrative creations* are processes in which their drug use can be viewed from the 'inside' as 'normal human behaviour', particularly with regard to the recreational use of drugs (Skirrow 1993:194), and as a 'mainstream phenomenon' (Henderson 1993:128); the latter issue has come to the fore in recent studies in the drugs field and is of particular relevance to women sufferers who use drugs (Taylor 1993).

Gender and the narrative

This brings us to a discussion of our second interest: to demonstrate how the narrative operates through a gender-sensitive lens. Narratives of ill health tend to focus on the self viewed in relation to its past. The effect on one's reconstituted past is twofold: 'this past', as a temporal, spatial component of one's history, is located or embodied in time (Robinson 1990) and 'this past' becomes reconstructed or interpreted 'in the present' (i.e. narrative construction) as having a purpose and 'accounting for present disruptions' – adding a 'teleological component' to one's biography (Williams 1984:178). We contend that, from the vantage point of gender, a conception of narrative construction must consider the gendered process involved. The question here is: how is gender embedded in narratives of ill health and, specifically, psychotropic drug use?

In answering this question, three key concerns must be considered: the temporal context of the narrative; what this narrative reconstruction signifies; and, furthermore, how 'misfortune' is perceived within this reconstruction. First, the narrative must be recognised as being located within a gendered, social order over and above a temporal context. Similar to men's narratives, women's narratives deal with the relationship between the self and society. However, within a temporal context, women's narratives differ. This is because, in contrast to men's, women's narratives expose 'women's condition and the collective representations of women as they have been shaped by society' – beyond the temporal context of individual women's biographies (Chanfrault-Duchet 1991:78). In the drugs field, insights into women's conditions, the collective representations of women's drug-taking behaviour, and the gendered character of these conditions and representations have liberating possibilities which have only just begun to come to the surface (Bepko 1991; Sargent 1992; Ettorre 1992; Hafner 1992; Taylor 1993).

Second, one must examine critically the notion of the narrative construction of ill health from the point of view of what it signifies. For example, in his accounts of chronic illness, Williams (1984) argues rightly, in our view, that the reconstructed narrative signifies key reference points in an individual's unfolding, historical relationship between the body, the self and society. But, through a gender-sensitive lens, there are observable differences in how femininity and masculinity can be inscribed on the body by the self in interaction with society (Holland *et al.* 1993). Also, illness experiences for women tend to be conceptualised in and through the culture of medicine, pushing women more than men – even those women with healthy bodies – into spaces of ill health, particularly with regard to child-bearing (Graham and Oakley 1991).

Third, if we speak about how individuals perceive misfortunes, as Williams (1984) does, we need to recognise the workings of gender within this process. For example, for women, the genesis of their misfortunes (i.e. health-related or otherwise) may stem from their actual experiences of being women (Graham 1990). Alternatively, men's misfortunes may stem from their collective need to be bearers of the 'patriarchal mode' in society (Heath 1987) or their refusal, if not compunction, to do so. If we focus our attention on the narratives of long-term psychotropic drug users, we see an added dimension: their experiences of misfortune are embodied within their drug-taking experiences (Montagne 1991), seen as proceeding from any number of tragedies, life difficulties, mental health conditions or anxiety states. In this context, a thus far unanswered question arises: How does masculinity or femininity affect one's experience of long-term drug taking as an embodiment of misfortune?

Narratives, specifically narratives of chronic illness, may provide key reference points to an evolving connection between the body and the meaning of illness, sufferers and the social organisation of their worlds and the strategies they use in adapting to society. Nevertheless, constructing narratives of long-term psychotropic drug use must provide a framework for understanding the multi-dimensional emergence of life stories – lives embedded in a society whose 'master narrative' is all about preserving class, gender and race as appropriate social and subjective categories of disadvantage. How drug users' lives unfold within this master narrative, shaping their own personal narratives, will be our focus in the following discussions in this chapter.

THE STUDY OF LONG-TERM USE OF PSYCHOTROPICS

Our study focused on long-term psychotropic drug use and gender-related factors contributing to the initiation, continuation and termination of use. At this stage in the discussion, it is important for the reader to have a clear methodological picture of this study. First, we will provide an overview of our respondents. Next, we proceed to a full discussion of our data collection measures. Then we offer a description of our respondents by type of user, drugs used, and frequency and length of use.

The target population were adults who were using, or had used, tranquillisers and hypnotics, and who were living in a metropolitan area of southern Finland. The aim was to recruit 50 men and 50 women for a questionnaire survey and to select 10 people from among the respondents for interview.

The study population was recruited in two ways – through local health care centres and through newspapers between January and April 1992. Primary care physicians offered the questionnaire to patients who were users of minor tranquillisers and who had entered the health care system through a municipal health centre, a voluntary health centre or an alcohol treatment centre. Forty-eight subjects (30 men and 18 women) were recruited in this way.

The recruitment of respondents through newspapers involved two phases. During the first phase, journalists summarised the aim of the planned study in the local newspapers and provided a telephone number so that people could volunteer. In the second phase, an advertisement was placed in a local newspaper to recruit people who were users or who had used minor tranquillisers. This recruitment method yielded 52 people – 13 men and 39 women.

Table 6.1 Distribution of the study population by recruitment site and gender

Recruitment site	Males	Females	Total
Health care centres	(30)	(18)	(48)
Municipal health centres	1	4	5
Voluntary health centres	–	2	2
Alcohol treatment centres	29	12	41
Newspapers	(13)	(39)	(52)
Phase 1: Story	9	31	40
Phase 2: Advertisement	4	8	12
Total	43	57	100

Table 6.1 shows that women were more inclined to volunteer through the advertisement in the newspaper, whereas the majority of the men (30 out of 43) were recruited through health care centres – in particular, alcohol treatment centres. The skewed distribution of the respondents by recruitment site and gender was unexpected and at the same time was an indicator of the gendered character of long-term psychotropic drug use.

The final study population consisted of 43 men and 57 women (three men and seven women were selected for future interview). The average age for the total sample was 51.8 and was lower for males (46.2) than females (56.1). (See Table 6.2.)

Table 6.2 Distribution (%) of study population by age, employment status, civil status and place of residence

	Females	Males	Total
Average age	56.1	46.2	51.8
Employment status			
Retired	63	28	48
Employed	21	32	26
Unemployed	11	35	21
Other	3	5	4
Housewife	2	0	1
Civil status			
Married	40	32	37
Separated or divorced	23	37	29
Unmarried	10	21	15
Widowed	18	5	12
Living together	9	5	7
Residence			
Suburb	51	49	50
City centre	28	40	33
Other	21	11	17
Total (%)	100	100	100
N	57	43	100

Almost half the respondents were retired, which explains the higher proportion of female (63 per cent) to male (28 per cent) respondents. While a third of male respondents and a fifth of female respondents were employed, a much higher proportion of males (35 per cent) than females (11 per cent) were unemployed. The category housewife was not particularly common. As other research has shown, housewives, in comparison with employed women in Finland, do not have a higher rate of psychotropic drug use, although this is the case in the other Nordic countries (Riska *et al.* 1993). With regard to current or former occupation, 84 per cent of the respondents were, or had been, involved in lower white-collar or blue-collar occupations. Overall, 44 per cent of the respondents were living with a partner, either married or not. Males reported more often than females that they were separated or divorced, while females more often than males were widowed. Half of all respondents lived in the suburbs, while a third lived in the inner city area. It should be noted that these social background characteristics are representative of users in the larger Finnish population (Riska *et al.* 1993).

The survey included 35 questions, of which 11 provided social background information about the respondent. Eleven questions assessed the respondents' drug habits. Psychotropic drug use was measured by the question: 'Do you currently use tranquillisers or sleeping pills?' *Current users* were defined as those who responded that they had: (a) used such drugs regularly or fairly regularly during the past month; and (b) used such drugs a couple of times during the past month. *Ex-users* were those who were not at present using tranquillisers or sleeping pills but who had used such drugs in the past regularly at least during a month.

The characteristics of the respondents' drug use were measured by types of drug used, number of drugs used, frequency of use and length of use. Initially, the study aimed at focusing only on users of minor tranquillisers. As the analysis of data progressed, it became evident that the respondents had listed major tranquillisers in addition to the 36 minor tranquillisers in the appendix to the questionnaire. Concerning types of drug used, the final list of coded drugs included 36 minor tranquillisers (benzodiazepines, i.e. hypnotics and sedatives) and 28 other psychotropics (mainly neuroleptics and antidepressants). In terms of drugs used, respondents were divided into three categories:

1 pure minor tranquilliser user, i.e. used only minor tranquillisers;
2 mixed user, i.e. used both minor or major tranquillisers and other psychotropics;
3 pure major tranquilliser user, i.e. used only major tranquillisers.

The mechanisms of introduction to drug use were measured by self-assessed reasons for drug use, type of prescribing physician, and role of the lay referral network (i.e. acquaintances, friends, relatives). The mechanisms of continuation and/or termination were assessed by questions concerning difficulties experienced in terminating drug use, desire to stop use, raising the issue of terminating drug use with the prescribing physician as well as others, and the physician's and the lay person's reactions to the desire to stop drug use. Ten questionnaire respondents (seven women and three men) were interviewed. These interviews are used as the basis for personal narratives.

The use of psychotropics

A majority of the drug users were current users (85 per cent), while the remainder were ex-users (15 per cent). There were, however, marked gender differences between the current users and the ex-users: 19 per cent of female and 7 per cent of male respondents were ex-users (see Table 6.3).

In terms of drugs used, females were, to the same extent as males, pure minor tranquilliser (i.e. hypnotics and sedatives) users and mixed users, but males were slightly more often than females users of only major tranquillisers (i.e. neuroleptics and antidepressants). The latter finding appears to be related to the alcohol habits of male respondents. These habits and male and female users' dependency on alcohol will be discussed in Chapter 8.

A majority reported that they had used more than two drugs either consecutively or one after the other. Female users reported this more often than their male counterparts. The most frequently used drugs were: Oxepam (oxazepam), by 16 per cent of respondents; Halcion (triazolam), by 7 per cent; Diapam (diazepam), by 6 per cent; Mogadon (nitrazepam), by 4 per cent; Insomin (nitrazepam), by 4 per cent and Temesta (lorazepam), by 4 per cent.

A majority of the respondents reported that they used their drugs daily, with more females reporting this than males (see Table 6.3). As many as 20 per cent had used some kind of psychotropic drug for over 15 years. The average length of time for use of these drugs was nine years, and was higher for female users (11.4 years) than for male users (6.1 years).

Table 6.3 Distribution (%) of drug users by type of user, drug used, number of drugs used, length and frequency of use

	Females	Males	Total
Type of user			
Current user	81	93	85
Ex-user	19	7	15
Type of drug used			
Pure minor tranquilliser user	44	42	43
Mixed user	47	44	46
Pure major tranquilliser user	9	14	11
Number of drugs used			
One drug	19	28	23
Two drugs	23	30	26
Three drugs	18	16	17
Four drugs	19	10	15
Five or more	21	16	19
Length of drug use			
<1 year	3	19	10
1–<3 years	16	26	20
3–<6 years	9	9	9
6–<16 years	30	25	28
16–<26 years	16	7	12
26 years or +	10	5	8
No answer	16	9	13
Frequency of use			
Daily	67	57	63
Sometimes during a week	27	17	23
Less than once a week	4	17	9
Did not remember	2	9	5
Total (%)	100	100	100
N	57	43	100

The above discussion has attempted to provide a full methodological picture of our study. In the following discussions, we will highlight key theoretical concepts which we see as important in understanding the lives of long-term psychotropic drug users and apply these concepts to the subjective accounts of our respondents.

Long-term use: personal narratives

In looking at the personal narratives of our respondents, we examine specifically their stated health-related reasons for psychotropic drug use as well as key temporal occurrences or life events related to this use. These narratives reveal how gender as a social institution has shaped the narrators' drug-taking lives. Women's narratives are embedded in an awareness of internal stressors or psychological distress, such as depression or tiredness, impinging on female bodies. Their drug use reflects a somewhat vulnerable state of mental health and the need for internal well-being. While revealing a certain level of psychological distress, men's narratives tend to be characterised by external stressors or exogenous agents (e.g. pressure of work or work responsibilities), which thrust masculine bodies into a state of tension. Their drug use reflects physical release as a goal towards a state of social and psychological well-being. Here a gendered distinction is evident. On the one hand, there is a distinction between distress or depression and mental health – a distinction viewed as crucial analytically in building a gender-sensitive framework on health (Pugliesi 1992). On the other hand, this distinction implies that, in recounting the genesis of their misfortunes in a temporal context, women focus inwards, specifying the internal resources of feelings and emotions, while men's gaze is outwards, highlighting their responsibilities in the external world.

In explaining the intractability of their drug use, survey respondents reported health-related reasons, linked either to specific symptoms experienced or to psychiatric health problems. All the respondents went through a checklist of health problems related to their drug use. The majority were bothered by insomnia (81 per cent), depression (77 per cent), nervousness or tension (74 per cent), tiredness (71 per cent) and bad memory (57 per cent). Tiredness and depression were the two high-ranking symptoms for females (84 per cent and 80 per cent respectively), while for males insomnia (95 per cent) and nervousness or tension (78 per cent) ranked highly. Users' narratives illustrate these findings vividly and pinpoint how the narrator's discursive subjectivity is consistently intersected by the rhythm of drug using. Put simply, drug use is necessary because it helps to create a sense of routine and order in the experience of internal distress for women and external pressures for men.

One female respondent, a sufferer from arteriosclerosis, spoke about her 'basic' tiredness. While she herself was the instigator of her drug use, she says that it is easier for a woman to get these drugs. The implication is that she was 'believed by her doctor':

'I asked for sleeping pills [first Mogadon, then Pacisyn] because I had so much pain that I could not get to sleep. . . . The biggest disadvantage is this basic tiredness . . . I think it is easier for doctors to believe a woman than a man.'

(59-year-old retired dressmaker)

Here the narrator acknowledges the workings of the gender order *vis-à-vis* these drugs, but nevertheless privileges the necessity for them in her life, given her experience of emotional distress and physical pain owing to a prior illness.

Another female respondent had used three types of minor tranquilliser (one after the other) over nine years, and she describes how her depression was diagnosed by her doctor:

'First I had this major depression. I took depression medication for several years. Halcion was prescribed when I suddenly had to go to work very early in the morning and then I asked for them because I was scared of the following morning and then I did not sleep at all. The doctor's diagnosis was "heavily depressive" and some other things I can't remember now. As I said, I can't remember everything. . . . These [pills] take away your memory. . . . It is more acceptable for a woman to be ill because women, at least in a male society, are supposed to be weak. It is more

understandable – a man is not allowed to be weak.'
(47-year-old library assistant)

While the routinisation of the female narrator's work performance was involved here, the doctor's diagnosis of depression privileged internal distress and a subsequent sick label
(i.e. 'heavily depressive') which she saw as a sign of weakness.

As stated earlier, men experienced similar emotional
distress. But the inception of their use revolved around the
routinisation and ordering of work pressures with a temporal
focus on the external. Here a male sufferer from nervousness,
another high-ranking symptom for men, says:

'[I got this medication because] I had a stressful job and
could not sleep because of work . . . I thought about things
in the night. . . . It was also my opinion that I needed them.
This is why I asked for these drugs.'
(74-year-old retired insurance director, ex-user)

Another male respondent with insomnia says:

'I worked at a place where there were interruptions in the
night. During the night there were all kinds of things
happening and I could not get any sleep at all and I woke up
unnecessarily when I thought I heard the doorbell ring. At
that time, the kids were at the age when I had to wait for
them to come home at night. That is how my sleeping
problems started.'
(56-year-old porter)

But this male narrator reveals that routine and order did not
free him from the risk of disruption, and were also mitigated
by the values and assumptions of the doctor. This risk of
disruption in his external world concerned not only his work
performance but also how the drugs interfered with leisure
time, a contentious issue for this narrator. He says:

'Once I had been awake all night and was going on a
summer holiday for a week the following day with my
grandchildren. I asked the doctor about the drugs because I
felt they affected me in the morning, and my driving. The
doctor replied that it was better to take the sleeping pills
than to stay awake. I totally disagree with this. I know this

for sure . . . I know these pills affect my driving. (I have been driving for 37 years – partly as my job.) I argued for several years about this with my doctor and he said my pills have no effects in the morning. I'm sure I had them in me in the morning. . . . Maybe I am a bit sensitive to the side effects of medicines. . . . If you have been awake for several nights you cannot think clearly and you just believe the doctor.'

(56-year-old porter)

The majority of the survey sample (51 per cent) related their drug use to psychiatric health problems. Other reasons (some health related, some not) were: alcohol (20 per cent); work related (11 per cent); somatic health problems (9 per cent); problems with partner (7 per cent); and other (2 per cent). Responses in female narratives tended to be more specific and focused on psychiatric health problems. For example, female users revealed:

'I was so tired so I had a nervous breakdown. I just cried and cried.'

(72-year-old machine worker, ex-user)

'I have weak nerves . . . I am a very emotional person.'

(57-year-old teacher)

'I am a little bit neurotic. My mother always told me that when I was a kid . . . I get nervous easily.'

(47-year-old library assistant)

'I became mentally ill in 1984 . . . My diagnosis was at that time a "borderline case".'

(33-year-old part-time cleaner)

The last narrator described herself as 'a medicine gymnast', suggesting that she had to go through 'many twists and turns to get her medication right'.

In comparison with women, men's feelings were expressed in a more opaque way and emphasised external stressors rather than internal distress – an emphasis also confirmed by their doctors. Nevertheless, male responses could also be seen as reflecting psychiatric health problems but in a gendered context. While they needed to work to be psychologically healthy, they also felt that the reasons for not sleeping remained a mystery and should be sorted out. For example:

'I think that I have already been taking these medicines for too long. It is an unnatural sleep and there should be something else. No doctor has ever asked me why I did not sleep. That is something they could try.... Maybe I should be away from work for longer. I realise that my troubles are because I live at my workplace.... They should have sorted out the basic reasons for not being able to sleep. I am now in such a bad condition that I can no longer sleep well even at my summer cottage.'

(56-year-old porter)

In a similar vein, another male narrator says:

'When my hands became bad the doctor told me that I could not work. I sat and thought about it for a day and did not sleep at night at all. So the following morning, I started working. The doctor saw that I had been working when I went to see him. I asked him if we should treat my head or my hands. The doctor said, "We treat your hands".'

(66-year-old farmer)

These narratives confirmed that this kind of male shame resulted from an endogenous agent – work. Furthermore, doctors unwittingly helped to perpetuate this shame.

Thirty per cent of male and 11 per cent of female drug users gave alcohol as the main reason for using these drugs. Although none of those interviewed had used pills mainly because of alcohol problems, many reported that they were aware of, what they referred to as, 'mixed users'. Some reported that alcohol use could lead to the use of these pills (e.g. to help hangovers or to sleep better) and that they had friends and acquaintances who were mixed users.

Thirteen per cent of females reported that the main reason for using these drugs was a marital problem, while no male respondent reported such a problem as a main reason. These women used their pills to help them cope with difficult feelings arising from their marital problems. The responses are revealing and again offer evidence of the emphasis which women narrators place on emotional distress.

'I have . . . had difficulties with my marriage and I blame
him (my husband). . . . Now I have made it clear that I want
to live the rest of my life in peace, and I don't want to be
yelled at for any reason because I have tried the best I can in
this world.'

(57-year-old teacher)

One female respondent began using tranquillisers after her
father died and then began, after stops and starts, to become a
regular daily user because of problems with her husband.
Later on her narrative revealed that she had been a constant
victim of her husband's violence:

'Tensopam was given to me at the time of my father's death
. . . I just continued using them because they helped me in
certain situations. Frankly, my husband was a difficult
person. Then I had none left and I did not get new ones . . .
I had a small pause in the Mogadon use [she had already
switched to Mogadon], but my mother died. Then I
continued again. It was because of my husband . . . when I
caught him going out with another woman. He had been
doing that for two years regularly . . . I did suspect it. I just
did not realise it but I caught him out because of an
anonymous phone call. Then I had to take the sleeping
pills.'

(66-year-old chauffeuse, ex-user)

In the above narrative, catching one's husband going out with
another woman is clearly not a health-related reason for drug
use. However, looking closely at the narrative, one sees that
being a victim of male violence, experiencing a husband's
infidelity and living with a difficult person were, in the
opinion of this woman's doctor, sufficient reason to tranquillise her. While the diagnosis was anxiety and sleeplessness, the
woman experienced emotional distress caused by extreme fear
of this outside agent – her husband. But the genesis of her use
was emotional distress and pills were viewed as a resource,
enabling her to get through a difficult situation.

She continues:

'We were separated for seven and a half years. I lived in
constant fear because my husband said that he would

always follow me. . . . He beat me – my ribs have been broken and I still have a mark on my eye. No one stood up to him. Before he died when he asked me for the last time if he could come home, I said, 'Never.' After that he was never sober and he died . . . and it was easier for me. . . . He was always following me. Once I went to a nearby city to a party and a car followed me all the way. I did not recognise the driver. I was so scared that when I arrived I locked the doors. Then I recognised him. My husband had followed me all the way. The pills have helped me in these kinds of situation.'

LIFE EVENTS RELATED TO DRUG USE

Survey respondents were given a checklist of possible life events which could be related to their drug use. They reported illness (60 per cent), pressure at work (53 per cent) and economic troubles (53 per cent). Here, as in the earlier discussions, male more than female responses were linked in some way to external stressors (i.e. work). One male narrator talked about his experience of 'lumberjack disease' as propelling him into his 16-year Oxepam use:

'I had lumberjack disease which still bothers me. My fingers got numb and ached so that I could not sleep. That's why they [Oxepam] were given to me so that I could sleep at night and then I became addicted to them. If I did not take a pill, I could not sleep at all during the night. It is still that way now . . . I was still working then. My fingers are like hooks and they ache. It is caused by the chain saw.'

(66-year-old farmer)

Another male respondent spoke about how his pills had helped him to maintain a daily work routine related to his experience of pressure at work:

'You have to keep up the daily routine and you cannot sleep in the daytime and you have to get up in the morning at a certain time. When you have stayed awake for a couple of nights, your working capacity deteriorates.'

(74-year-old retired insurance director, ex-user)

In contrast to male respondents who related their drug use to work, female respondents viewed their own illnesses as a key temporal awareness, directly related to their use of pills:

'I have been able to sleep for some periods, but when I got these bad knees and all the operations.... It was one year to three years ago . . . I was in surgery four times. After that I used pills all the time . . . I have had bad knees and all these allergies. . . . I get pills from the health centre doctor and from a specialist who takes care of my knees. I ask for them when I need more.'

(57-year-old teacher)

Another female respondent:

'First came the glandular problem, then the sleeping problem, and then age. At this age you have to consider everything. If you are 30 years old, your situation is totally different from mine.'

(51-year-old postal worker)

What is interesting in the above is that, whether we look at health reasons for use or key life events, there are gender differences. This was seen in users' own perceptions and ephemeral awareness: work was established as a key temporal marker for men, while for women the onset of physical illness acted as a signifier of the need for psychotropic drug taking. These findings confirm the notion that, within the context of chronicity, there are clear gender differences in the perception of the characteristics of stressors – an issue which was illustrated in Chapter 4.

In conclusion, we have attempted in this chapter to provide an insider's perspective on long-term psychotropic drug use. Additionally, we have exposed how the workings of gender can indeed affect the genesis of a sufferer's drug use. In the following chapter, we turn our attention to the group level of analysis in the social construction of psychotropic drug use and extend our attempt to maintain the status of users as speaking subjects.

Chapter 7

Gendered moods and the lay culture

INTRODUCTION

In the preceding chapter, we focused on the individual layer of analysis in the social construction of psychotropic drug use. Through the use of narratives, we attempted to preserve long-term users' discursive subjectivity by allowing them to speak as subjects. This discursive subjectivity was analysed from a gender-sensitive perspective. Building on this perspective and our theoretical framework presented in Chapter 4, this chapter focuses the reader's attention on the group level of analysis in the social construction of psychotropic drug use. The overall aim of the chapter is twofold. First, we shed additional light on lay concerns which should be explored in understanding long-term psychotropic drug use. Second, we offer a picture of users which is outside the social vacuum in which they have been traditionally portrayed.

In examining this group level of analysis, we look first at what constitutes normal moods and 'nerves' in the non-professional setting; how bodies are disciplined in the discourse on stress and nerves; and where psychotropic drug use fits into this picture.

WHAT CONSTITUTES NORMAL MOODS AND 'NERVES' IN THE LAY CULTURE?

Individuals who use psychotropic drugs define themselves, and are defined by others, as those who experience 'nerves' and therefore somatise their 'stress'. Feeling guilty or ashamed, they have not been able to resolve their 'conflicts of living'. These conflicts, personal struggles evidenced by their use of drugs, are between themselves as sufferers from 'nerves' and their stressful lifestyles. Besides having this sort of inner logic about the state of their moods, psychotropic drug users are aware of the social and cultural representations of their drug use in the form of lay idioms. For example, 'Too much stress is unhealthy'; 'Somatising stress can cause even more stress for a sufferer'; 'People with nerves need to learn how to cope with their changing moods'. These lay idioms are drawn from existing social values; are shared by others; stem from the social surroundings in which sufferers live and form the basis of generalised reactions to psychotropic drug taking in the lay culture. The lay culture structures this discourse on 'nerves' and 'stress' as states needing control or at least containment in an individual's quest for health (Mullen 1994).

HOW ARE BODIES DISCIPLINED IN THE LAY DISCOURSE ON STRESS AND NERVES?

The most visible social values which the lay culture draws upon are discipline and order. For example, achieving and maintaining a healthy body and mind requires discipline and order. Health and well-being imply discipline both in terms of the maintenance of one's health and one's occupational work. In order to be seen as healthy, one needs to order one's health, social behaviour and one's body as being congruent with cultural representations of health. Here the body is perceived as one of a worker, a concept underscoring the significance of maintaining a healthy body for the performance of one's work duties and responsibilities. Of course, this has specific gender implications, given that images of the working body shift and, furthermore, are contextualised by cultural notions of masculinity and femininity. Simply, conceptions about working bodies are gendered with the notion of work tending to be linked to male bodies, not female bodies. This should not be surprising, given that the ethics of health are masculine and the working role is an operational definition of health and masculinity for men.

WHERE DOES PSYCHOTROPIC DRUG USE FIT INTO THIS PICTURE?

In societies governed by the social values of order and dis-cipline, drug taking puts a strain on these values and working bodies because all drug use appears as 'counter to the ethos of a disciplinary society' (Smart 1984:34). Drug taking is not viewed as an admirable way of adapting to the stresses and strains of modern life. Drug taking is a sign of a weakened self, unable to adapt to 'nerves'. On a cultural level, it is perceived as a value strain in itself – an unwanted social stress, symbolic of an uncoveted vigour which exerts undue pressure on the social order. It strains the common or lay stock of understanding about what constitutes social well-being, healthy bodies and an acceptable quality of life. It creates cultural dissonance within this common stock of understanding. Therefore, lay idioms on what are acceptable and respectable 'nerves' for healthy bodies do not fit comfortably with psychotropic drug use.

CULTURAL DISSONANCE AND SOCIAL VALUES VIS-À-VIS DRUG TAKING

As we saw in the above discussion, discipline and order are viewed as ensuring the maintenance of a working society of healthy individuals. This notion is based on two interrelated views of social behaviour. First, health reflects self-control in a disciplinary society. Second, drug use is symbolic, as well as an indicator, of loss of self-control. While psychotropic drug use, on the individual level, may be experienced as a way of dealing with stress or nerves, the cultural representation of this behaviour is one in which a cultural strain or dissonance emerges between health, self-control and drug use. Let us now focus on key theoretical issues related to this cultural dis-sonance. In looking at these issues, we ask: 'How is health and, in turn, illness evaluated within the lay culture of "strain"?'

For Parsons (1958:165) illness, and in particular mental illness, was defined in terms of the extent to which the individual could meet the expectations of social roles and enter particular social relationships. Parsons regarded health and illness as universal categories while, at the same time, viewing them as socially and culturally relative categories. In the context of American society, health and illness were related to key values: activism, worldliness and instrumentalism. On the basis of these values, illness became a problem with an individual's capacity for achieving his or her goals and self-fulfilment. These values seem, today, to permeate Western culture and increasingly to be used by society as well as individuals as markers for qualifying them for full membership in society. Activism is a measure and, at the same time, a consequence of being in control of one's life.

Here the value of self-control as an indicator of health emerges clearly. As Crawford (1984) suggests: 'Healthy behaviour has become a moral duty and illness an individual failing. . . . Health is a metaphor for self-control.' The value of health and hence self-control as a virtue is characterised by a cultural movement which Crawford (1980) calls 'healthism'. Healthism is pursued by individuals through health promotion behaviours and supported by current neo-liberal health policies which are touting lifestyle politics as the panacea whereby the public health of the population will be improved.

In Crawford's view, those seen to be pursuing their health demonstrate their participation in a 'rite of belonging' to a disciplined, well-ordered society. Those who have not performed this ritual (e.g. those using drugs and, therefore, not possessing self-control) are not only excluded from society but also appear to fall under the purview of what Armstrong (1983:10) calls 'the epidemiological gaze': a gaze which helps to shift concerns of social hygiene and public health from 'the environment to the mode of transmission between people and to ramifications of social relationships'. For example, drug users, within the framework of discipline, facilitate the proliferation of the epidemiological gaze into the social arena. Appearing as those who have not performed this rite of belonging, they help to shift both public health and lay concerns from a focus on the environment to one on the ramifications of their drug-using behaviour on social relationships. While the epidemiological gaze emphasises the mode of transmitting diseases (including social diseases such as drug use) between people, the emphasis is primarily individualistic. Translated into the lay culture, these ideas suggest that the drug user does not belong to a healthy society and his or her behaviour is evaluated in an individualistic manner – in terms of what is normal behaviour for a healthy individual.

In this aura of individualism, drug use – whether legal or illegal – is viewed as a measure of an individual's incapacity to meet the criteria of functional adequacy in society. Therefore, despair, stress and anxiety are operational signs of not being in control of one's life. While psychotropic drug use, on the individual level, may be experienced as a way of dealing with stress or nerves, the cultural representation of this behaviour is one in which the drug user is viewed as someone whose life is controlled, if not ruled or governed totally, by drug taking. Hence, the drug user is not in control of his or her life; the drugs have taken over control. This cultural representation derives from an all-pervasive cultural belief: self-control is the key to the orderly flow of social life. Drug users do not adhere to the norm of exerting self-control. Put simply, they cannot 'stick' within society because they do not have that necessary social glue: self-control.

In this context, Waldorf and his colleagues aptly state, with special reference to American society:

> In a deeply Protestant culture rooted in the individualism of 'self-made' men and women, self-control has always been the social glue of society. . . . A cursory comparison of licit and illicit drugs shows little relationship between the dangers or social costs of a drug and its legal status.
>
> (Waldorf *et al.* 1991:5–7)

THE ORGANISATION OF UNCOMFORTABLE MOODS AND DESPAIR WITHIN THE LAY CULTURE

As highlighted in the above discussion, stress, nerves or feelings of despair are signs of not being in control. These symptoms intrude upon the lay culture as being emblematic of illness and ill-being. They disrupt social relationships, and, at the same time, are viewed as disorders and personal misfortunes, entering the lives of previously healthy individuals.

Uncomfortable moods hamper self-control. But this cultural definition of adequacy – self-control – has far-reaching implications for women. Women's structural position, as shaped by the gender system, makes them perpetually unfit to meet the general, cultural norm of adequacy. Women seldom have control over their lives to the extent that men do. Within the context of prevailing male values, self-control for women appears rarely, if ever, as an achievable goal. In this sense, women's disciplinary efforts are valued less than men's. As society's emotional and health workers, women, in the context of the traditional lay culture, appear as the primary carriers of stress and thus prime targets for psychotropic drug use.

Men have always seemed to have the 'edge' on rationality. Furthermore, the idea of men as both the possessors and dispensers of reason and hence self-control is embedded within our culture. Historically, this idea fixes any semblance of loss of control, irrationality and, ultimately, madness as a female malady (Showalter 1985; Chesler 1989). Thus, women emerge inevitably as being somehow deviant or 'out of order' within this overall lay culture of self-control.

If 'sufferers' from stress (particularly women) alleviate their symptoms through psychotropic drug use, they support implicitly a traditional biomedical belief: pharmacological aids to relieve anxiety and depression are worthwhile because they have been used throughout history. This idea of the functional universality of psychoactive substances becomes translated into the lay culture of stress and, in turn, asserts that these drugs have more positive than negative effects in controlling both 'unwanted' symptoms and so social behaviour. But that women more than men sufferers are seen to experience the need for these effects tends to be either irrelevant or minimised.

Furthermore, when women do become involved with these drugs, they are seen to have a greater problem and to be more psychologically disturbed than their male counterparts (Broom and Stevens 1991). This demonstrates the power of the male value, self-control and the intractability of women's use of these drugs.

In terms of this intractability of women's use, few authors have considered whether or not there are any socially beneficial reasons for, what one author refers to as, the 'dulling of the female mind through prescribed drugs'. Here, Dworkin, elucidates clearly:

> The dulling of the female mind is neither feared nor noticed; nor is the loss of vitality or independence . . . the female is valued for looks and domestic, sex and reproductive work, none of which requires that she be alert. She is given drugs because nothing is lost when she is drugged. . . . She is given drugs because she is not much valued.
>
> (Dworkin 1983:158)

But, in the context of the above discussion, how are uncomfortable moods organised through non-professional channels? Here the lay response to 'stress' or uncomfortable moods implies the mobilisation of a variety of non-professional channels, including working through significant others, using lay alternatives or self-help to alleviate the sufferer's symptoms.

THE ORGANISATION OF NON-PROFESSIONAL CHANNELS

In an attempt to make visible sufferers' involvement in different social spaces within the lay culture, the following discussion focuses on lay referral networks and how, within these networks, individuals are introduced to psychotropic drug taking. We also examine the issue of self-help groups as a lay alternative to psychotropic drug taking and users' perceptions of this alternative. Finally, we offer a brief picture of the types of lay remedy besides medications that users value and employ in dealing with stress. As in the previous chapter, narrative material as well as survey data will be used to illustrate these key areas.

Lay referral networks and the role of significant others

Help-seeking behaviour begins in most cases with a casual exploration of diagnosis and remedies with significant others. This lay referral network consists of non-professionals, such as family members, friends or acquaintances, who assist individuals in interpreting their symptoms and in recommending a course of action (Freidson 1960; McKinlay 1973; Scambler *et al.* 1981). The picture that emerges from our empirical work reveals that lay referral networks provided a significant channel for sufferers in their introduction to psychotropic drugs. For example, the majority of users had been introduced to a 'psychotropic drug-using culture' through their relatives, friends or acquaintances. A majority of both male and female users said that these significant others had used psychotropics regularly for a long time (see Table 7.1). As Table 7.1 shows, this lay referral system constituted the main channel of introduction to psychotropic drug use for slightly over a quarter (26 per cent) of our survey respondents.

Table 7.1 Distribution (%) of psychotropic drug users by the extent of use and sharing of psychotropics by significant others

	Females	Males	Total
Long-term usage among significant others			
Yes	61	51	57
No	16	23	19
Don't know	23	26	24
Received drugs from significant others			
Yes	20	35	26
No	80	65	74
Total (%)	100	100	100
N	57	43	100

There was a marked gender difference in the non-professional introduction to psychotropic drug use. While a fifth of the female users reported that they had initially received their drugs from friends, acquaintances or relatives, as many as a third of male respondents reported this channel of introduction. These findings indicate that male users are often introduced to the psychotropic drug culture by significant others, most likely women, who openly share their drugs and initiate them into pill taking. One sees here a type of gender role reversal, if we compare this finding with previous ones in the related field of illegal drug use. There, a consistent finding is that women heroin users are initiated into heroin use by men (Hser *et al.* 1987). In contrast, our finding suggests that women, rather than men, may be the pushers in the 'tranx-using culture'. Additionally, 'tranx pushing' appears to be mainly carried out in the private, household domain where a woman giving drugs to her partner may be perceived as an extension of her caring role.

On a related level, as Miles' (1988) study showed, women play a strategic role in this process of lay advice to other women with regard to feelings of 'not coping' or 'sleeplessness'. Furthermore, Graham (1984) and Stacey (1988) have highlighted women's crucial role as the primary health workers in the informal sector of health care. This role implies, however, that women share not only their 'labour of love' but also their remedies with others. In the context of our empirical study, women users appeared, in this way, as likely to introduce unwittingly other women and men into psychotropic drug use. As previous research has revealed (Horowitz 1977), men are more hesitant than women in seeking professional psychiatric help. Women are most likely to have a major role in diagnosing men's psychiatric symptoms as well as finding medical remedies in the lay system of care.

In addition, in the broader context of women as health workers in both the non-professional setting and the professional system of care, some women have organised their concerns within a social movement. Here the emergence of a women's health movement as a recognisable, collective endeavour has been documented in the United States (Ruzek 1976; Mellow 1989) and Britain (Doyal 1981, 1983; O'Sullivan 1987). But women-centred initiatives have been surprisingly few in the area of psychotropic drugs.

This discussion about users' introduction to psychotropic drug use by non-professional channels suggests that the lay referral network plays an important role in introducing sufferers to psychotropics. There are distinct, gendered structures influencing patterns of drug use: women in their capacity as health workers in an informal system of health care serve as initiators of use. Men tend to be the passive recipients in this initiation process.

Self-help groups as a lay alternative to psychotropic drug use

The discussion about medicalisation (Zola 1972) has over the past decade spurred lay initiatives in health, and self-help groups have become viable options to the hierarchical structure of and authority implicit in modern medicine (Katz 1981). In the literature on psychotropic drug use, self-help groups, as an alternative to psychotropic drug use (particularly minor tranquillisers), have been identified as a key issue within the informal system of health care (Ettorre 1986). Self-help groups and local community groups, organised with professional social workers' support, can be viable alternatives to psychotropic drug use (Ettorre 1986; Hatfield 1987). With the expansion of drug services in Britain in the early 1980s, there was a growing interest in organised tranquilliser support groups as well as government-funded tranquilliser agencies (MacGregor et al. 1992).

The existence of these groups has revealed the gendered character of this type of help-seeking behaviour (Melville 1984; Haddon 1984; Curran and Golombok 1985; Trickett 1991; Jerome 1991; Ettorre 1992). Additionally, some enlightened professionals, located on the boundaries of this lay system of care, have appeared as self-help advocates (Hamlin and Hammersley 1989a, 1989b, 1990; Hatfield 1987; Women's National Commission 1988).

In our empirical study, the issue of self-help emerged primarily within the context of user narratives. Here it should be noted that, at the time of our study, there were no self-help groups for psychotropic drug users within users' localities, although one group was in an early stage as we shall see below.

Looking at the narratives as a whole, one sees that users had varying ideas and feelings concerning the benefits, or indeed the usefulness, of self-help groups for them on a subjective level. Their knowledge about the existence of (in other localities), or their perceived lay need for, these groups was also divergent. Nevertheless, the concept of self-help had a general appeal, regardless of the fact that some users had never heard of these groups before, while others had. What can be gleaned from these narratives are the positive meanings and social 'flavour' that self-help groups had in the minds, if not experiences, of users. This was generally true for both males and females. In terms of this contextualised experience, self-help groups were viewed primarily as a 'beneficial' or 'good' lay alternative to drug taking. In terms of treatment or rehabilitation, our group of long-term users appeared to be more familiar with the options within the formal health care system than the lay culture. Nevertheless, many seasoned users perceived self-help groups as a 'viable way' of easing them into a more supportive and less isolated informal system of care. From a gender perspective, this lay setting offered the opportunity of 'sharing feelings' with others similar to themselves – an opportunity which was found to be particularly attractive for female long-term users.

Let us look first at the narratives of those who had never heard of self-help groups. One female user, who said she was extremely nervous, was eager to consider the possibility of what a self-help group could provide for her. In her view, self-help groups, 'where everyone would be like me', would be 'wonderful' because she would feel released from feelings of guilt. This narrator also revealed that she needed help and, interestingly enough, one form of help seeking, in her view, was to respond to enquiries about our study. She said:

'It [a self-help group] would be interesting and a good alternative for me. I now feel so guilty and the fault is totally in myself. When I don't cheer up, it has to do with my nerves. I have to feel good before I can go anywhere or have hobbies or do something. . . . It does not help to worry, but I cannot let it go. . . . I have not discussed this with anyone, you see, except for the doctor and doctors give you drugs. I think it would be wonderful to become a member of a self-help group where everyone would be like me. That's why I answered this questionnaire in the first place, so I could get some help or talk to someone. . . . I have no one to talk to and I don't want to bore my friends with my problems.'

(57-year-old teacher)

Another woman user, whose husband continually referred to her as 'an addict', felt initially that self-help groups might help her, but she had reservations. Her qualms were not about her potential participation in a self-help group but rather about the proximity of a meeting place for this type of group. This was because she felt 'stress' if she had to travel further than 10 kilometres from her home and the local city was at a distance of 15 kilometres. Nevertheless, in her final analysis, the idea of participating in such a group was perceived positively. She said:

'In a way that [a self-help group] might help me, but if it is in [local city], it is too far away for me. It would just give me stress. . . . If there were a group somewhere close to where I live, I would definitely go.'

(51-year-old postal worker)

In a similar vein, others who had not heard of self-help groups also had positive notions or ideas about their worth. For example:

'It would certainly be good to belong to a self-help group. Groups are always good no matter what kind of a group. You get to talk.'

(59-year-old female retired dressmaker)

'I have never heard of [self-help groups]. But a great many of my friends have . . . maybe it has something to do with the age that we live in that we all have our problems. So we have discussed these things. I suppose that's a kind of self-help group of our own and we are both men and women. But, of course, to belong to a group would be good, but I cannot say if it would help me to stop using Temesta. I think I have to stop using it by myself.'

(47-year-old female library assistant)

One rather isolated woman user had been shunned by her friends because she took psychotropic drugs. Early on in her

drug-taking career, her friends saw her as 'needing psychological treatment'. They therefore thought that she was 'crazy'
or 'mad' because she 'took these drugs'. Now she was something of an outsider in her social circle. She believed that a
self-help group would be beneficial, given that she had already experienced a narrowing lay channel of support as well
as a diminished friendship network as a result of her drug
taking. She contemplated:

> 'A self-help group would be a good idea. Yes, it could be
> good. . . . For those of us, like myself, who are very shy, a
> group would help. Maybe we would open up. When I first
> started my medication no one said anything to me [about
> alternatives]. I didn't talk about them [pills] either . . .
> because at the time people considered you mad if you took
> them. . . . Nowadays you can talk about these things. But
> then no one talked to me or tried to help me. Now you can
> talk more openly.'
>
> (72-year-old retired machine worker)

Like the above female narrator, the life of the following male
user also reflected a deep sense of isolation. He was uncertain,
if not sceptical, as to the worth of these groups for himself.
Within his contextual knowledge of himself and his drug
taking, he wondered what the 'gain' would be for him. As a
secret user, he felt 'ashamed' and tended to hide the extent of
his drug taking from others, apart from his family. If someone
were to ask him about his drug use, he believed he would, in
theory at least, reveal his 'secret'. Here it is interesting how, for
this narrator, the issue of self-help groups is linked implicitly
with the ability to disclose one's drug taking more publicly,
beyond the family. But there was a significant issue here: this
user's significant others (i.e. his family) did not know that he
was a *daily* user:

> 'I have not heard of self-help groups and I really wonder
> what would be in it for me. I tend to hide it [my use]. But I
> wouldn't hide it if someone were to ask me about it. I have
> two daughters – wonderful people both of them. They
> know that I take sleeping pills, but I have said that I do not
> take them all the time. Although I take them every night one

would think that a man who works would sleep all night. Somehow I am ashamed of it.'

(66-year-old farmer)

Another male user was ambivalent about whether or not he had ever heard of self-help groups. What is interesting here is that shame, which was experienced by the former male narrator, is a feeling which is actively and apparently successfully shunned by this narrator. Nevertheless, while there is a contrast between the two stories, this narrator has a further ambivalence surrounding the issue of men's, as opposed to women's, appropriate use of these drugs. Significantly, this narrator appears to imply that the use of self-help groups is more to do with conceptions about stopping use than personal disclosure of use. In this sense, the narrator reveals his bias towards a professional rather than a lay solution to his 'problem'.

'I might have heard about self-help groups but I cannot say whether or not I have . . . I just don't think that it is a problem stopping when you realise that it is not necessary to take [these drugs]. When a doctor or psychologist or whoever explains to you that these drugs are not necessary, I understand the reasons. Of course, it is another thing if you are working. Then it is rational to use sleeping pills. Doctors could warn about using too much. I don't think there is anything to be ashamed of, especially with sleeping pills. A man should not be more ashamed than a woman – even if you are a man and ask for these drugs. As long as you don't have serious psychiatric problems and have to go to a psychiatrist, there is nothing to be ashamed of. There is nothing to be ashamed of if you cannot get to sleep.'

(74-year-old retired insurance director)

Those users who had heard about self-help groups showed variations in the desired level of participation in these groups, if the opportunity arose. For example, one male user was familiar with the notion of self-help but was somewhat un-enthusiastic. His conceptual framework placed self-help groups in a moderately fixed setting. Simply, their main function was to help users stop using altogether. He envisaged his use of psychotropics in a temporal context. Therefore, he disclosed that he could do without self-help groups if they 'took a very long time' to get him off or were 'slow'. He felt that he had the 'courage' to come off on his own because he had done so with his dependence on nicotine. Nevertheless, a self-help group was provisionally, in this narrator's view, a positive option:

'I have heard about self-help groups. It might be a good alternative. I am such a busy person I don't know if it would suit me. If this group took a very long time and was slow, I can do without it. I know because I smoked for ten years and I found my own way to stop 23 years ago. (I tried to stop smoking several times but did not succeed.) At that time I smoked three packets a day. . . . But I found a good way to stop . . . I believe I have the courage that is needed to stop my drugs.'

(56-year-old porter)

A female, who seemed more enthusiastic than the above narrator, disclosed a certain level of emotional vulnerability. In the context of discussing self-help groups, she revealed how her psychotropic drug use began 20 years ago, when she was found to be infertile. At the time, she and her husband adopted a child. Discussing the issue of self-help had an emotional charge for this narrator. It triggered sensitive feelings about her drug career:

'Self-help groups would be good. I suppose they are a bit like Alcoholics Anonymous. You see, I do not know how I was so strong myself. I had used for 20 years. We adopted a boy then when I could not have a child of my own.'

(66-year-old chauffeuse)

In this context, another ex-user (female), our final narrator on self-help groups, disclosed that she was thinking of becoming involved in a self-help group. She revealed that there was a group for tranquilliser users being set up locally by her husband who, like herself, had a drug-taking career. Although she was currently an ex-user and received support in psycho-therapy, she said that she had consistently met other users 'to talk about her drug use' when she was still using. She revealed that the idea of setting up a support group came when she and her husband went to Germany. There they discovered, and were impressed by, a locally organised self-help group. This experience inspired her husband and motivated him to set up a group. She commented:

> 'When I think about these times of recession, it [a self-help group] would not compensate for my therapy but it [self-help] would be one form of help. I have noticed this myself that even if you don't have any formal groups [self-help groups] help. I know a lot of people who use and have used [tranquillisers] for a long time. When we meet and discuss our anxieties and other experiences, it is encouraging. You easily develop guilt feelings [when you are using] and you don't dare to talk about these things.'
>
> (33-year-old part-time cleaner)

In light of the above, there appeared to be a general consensus among users that self-help groups could be experienced subjectively as worthwhile or beneficial. Users recognised that self-help groups would enable them to feel less isolated and, perhaps, view themselves less as transgressors. Within the context of a self-help group, sufferers would be able to translate their personal experiences into a collective context with others who had suffered in similar ways. Also, gender differences in conceptions about help-seeking behaviour within the lay context of these respective groups emerged. The lay setting of the self-help group appeared to be focused more on self-disclosure for women than for men. Women welcomed the idea of sharing their experiences of uncomfortable moods with others. For example, sharing feelings with 'others like yourself' when you feel 'depressed', overwhelmed by 'nerves' or 'stress', was the salient focus within female user narratives. In addition, it was difficult for male narrators to consider the possibility of being in a self-help group without stopping drug use totally. Therefore, the lay idiom male users emphasised was stopping (e.g. 'total withdrawal') which, although appropriate in the self-help setting, is more of a reflection of professional than lay concerns. Although powerful emotions and feelings were apparent in men's narratives, they were not perceived as being either strong or sufficient enough for involvement in the self-help culture. Male narrators were less enthusiastic about bringing their personal experiences into the collective context of self-help groups. Their suffering was personal. Therefore, a male user, in the context of his drug-using career, needed some gain; disclosure in the context of the self-help group was not perceived as gain. Alternatively, in the context of their drug-using careers, women's desire for self-help and the lay idioms surrounding this desire appeared to be rooted in a sense of personal disclosure which would bring a sense of emotional well-being, a sense fostered within a group setting.

Use of other alternatives to medications as 'lay remedies'

In the following discussion, we provide an overview of the kinds of lay alternative to drugs which long-term psychotropic drug users have used. The picture that emerges locates users in a lay culture which confirms the value that individuals place on their health (Calnan 1987) and which, as suggested earlier in Chapter 4, provides the 'sufferer' with a series of structured actions to alleviate, if not eliminate, their 'problem', uncomfortable moods (i.e. stress, nerves, anxiety and depression). But this culture is also experienced as a fluid, social environment – a discursive space into which they are able to dip in order to receive needed support and resources. While being involved in long-term drug taking, some find that moving within this lay environment enables them to look for, as well as discover, viable options for coping with their lives without psychotropics. The options vary, as we shall see. However, most, if not all, lay alternatives are set within a framework where popular idioms dealing generally with stress and more particularly with psychotropic drug use form the basis of their actions. In turn, these actions have an ameliorative function, providing the user with a certain level of comfort and relief. When sufferers seek relief and comfort, lay alternatives appear as complements or supplements to their drug taking.

Sixty-one per cent of users employed lay alternatives in addition to drugs to ameliorate their symptoms. (See Table 7.2.) These included: exercise (43 per cent); alternative substances (36 per cent); relaxation (10 per cent); socialising (6 per

Table 7.2 Distribution (%) of drug users by use of 'lay' alternatives to ameliorate symptoms

	Females	Males	Total	
Use of 'lay' alternatives				
			%	N
Yes	56	67	61	61
No	44	33	39	39
Total (%)	100	100	100	100
N	57	43		
'Lay' alternatives used				
Exercise	38	48	43	26
Alternative substances	28	45	36	22
Relaxation	16	3	10	6
Socialising	12	0	6	4
Other	6	3	5	3
Total (%)	100	100	100	61
N	32	29		

cent) and other alternatives (e.g. reading and dieting) (5 per cent). The highest ranking lay alternative for both males and females was exercise. The use of alternative substances (including alcohol and natural or herbal remedies) ranked second as an alternative, but a higher percentage of male respondents (45 per cent) than female (28 per cent) reported the use of alternative substances. (Alcohol was the most prominent alternative substance for male users.) Many of the respondents (both male and female) who had used these lay alternatives discussed them in their narratives. One female narrator highlighted the variety of alternatives when she disclosed:

> 'I walk five kilometres every evening. . . . It has helped me to sleep better . . . going for a walk is a good outdoor al-
> ternative. To be outdoors a lot and make yourself exhausted in the evening. Even if sleep doesn't always come. . . . I also

had acupuncture for my headaches. It helped for a few weeks and then they started again . . . Massage I get all the time . . . You can get this in the countryside.'

(51-year-old postal worker)

Another female narrator told how she tried to relieve her stress:

'I take exercise and my form of exercise is dancing . . . belly-dancing . . . wonderful! Before . . . I did Greek dancing. . . . Belly-dancing is the only hobby I have had for a long time because I cannot sing any more, thanks to cigarettes.'

(47-year-old library assistant)

Relaxation exercises as well as acupuncture proved to be popular with some:

'I had acupuncture for migraine but it did not help. I have a relaxation cassette and it does make you sleepy. Then I don't need the pills . . . I take exercise as much as I can.'

(59-year-old dressmaker)

In this context, one male narrator reveals:

'I tried a relaxation course a long time ago . . . I could sleep at the time. But would it have helped anyway in a stressful situation? I tried it [this type of relaxation] for quite a long time . . . with books and cassettes. I could relax but if I had some thought that bothered me it did not help.'

(74-year-old retired insurance director)

Another male user who had heard of a herbal remedy, Valerian, through his lay referral network asked his doctor to help him obtain it:

'About a month ago I went to the doctor and asked for an alternative remedy and got Valerian. . . . It has no side effects. . . . It is a herbal remedy. . . . It feels really good and I do not feel anything in the mornings. . . . I have tried exercise. . . . I had acupuncture seven years ago for my headaches. . . . It did help.'

(56-year-old porter)

Two female users complained that some lay alternatives were

expensive in comparison with drugs. One of these users wanted to experiment with alternatives but the cost was prohibitive:

'They are expensive, all these alternatives . . . drugs are cheaper. . . . I would be prepared to try anything if only my headaches would go away and I could sleep – if the rest of my life was headache-free and I could sleep well. . . . Drugs are cheaper.'

(51-year-old postal worker)

Another female narrator who complained about the cost of some lay alternatives commented:

'I have thought about these alternatives but then there is the issue of money and all of them are expensive. I cannot afford them . . . but I use Imedeen [a fish protein preparation, marketed to women and claimed to make the skin look younger] . . . I started in the autumn when I had no lust for life because of the pain in my knees and my back. . . . When I had been taking Imedeen for two months all the aches went away. . . . I have not had to use any painkillers since then.'

(57-year-old teacher)

It is obvious from these excerpts that users employed a variety of lay alternatives to their medication. With few exceptions, they used these alternatives as a regularised form of 'personalised help-seeking behaviour'. Here, this visible help-seeking behaviour, based on the lay idiom, 'relief from stress', was not only organised practically as a desirable alternative to their drugs but also experienced contextually as a necessary diversion from psychotropic drug use. This appeared to be true regardless of the fact that some may have been using their drugs simultaneously. Here, lay alternatives appeared as both a complement and a supplement to psychotropic drug taking. In this way, their personalised help-seeking behaviour allowed them to structure their actions and give them some semblance of normality, if not stability, in their lives.

In conclusion, this chapter has focused on the group level of analysis in the social construction of psychotropic drug use. We have examined how sufferers with uncomfortable moods experience a sense of cultural dissonance, given the overriding social value – self-control. The gender implications of this cultural dissonance were highlighted. For example, in the light of the workings of the gender system, we saw that women more than men sufferers are subject to this social value and appear as perpetually unfit to meet the norm of adequacy. Furthermore, we looked specifically, with gender-sensitive eyes, at lay responses to uncomfortable moods including non-professional introduction to psychotropics, self-help groups as an alternative to drug taking and lay alternatives to medicines. The next chapter switches our current focus on non-professional settings to professional settings and examines how uncomfortable moods become structured into dependency and, in turn, a drug career.

Chapter 8

Dependency and the health care system

INTRODUCTION

The previous chapter focused on concerns directly related to users' involvement in the informal, lay system of care. This, the final chapter, looks at how dependency is organised into a drug career through the formal health care system. This system is viewed as comprising a 'diversity of segments: organisational (e.g. organisations of professionals and institutions), institutional (e.g. features of facilities and the interrelations between facilities), regulatory (e.g. such governmental agencies as the Food and Drug Administration), and financial (e.g. insurance and manufacturing)' (Brown 1989:291). This definition implies that, when looking at any segment within the health care system, one must provide links between these segments and what Brown sees as the 'deeper social structure of society'.

In this context, the reader will become aware that, on the one hand, the drug careers of users, shaped by involvement within the health care system, reflect a sharing of key, underlying themes: long-term users are dependent on psychotropic drug use and, through this type of dependence, they embark on a drug career. On the other hand, there are variations within these respective careers, as users confront different segments of the health care system. For example, sufferers vary in terms of age, race, ethnicity, social class, gender, able-bodiness and sexual orientation, and this affects how they make their way through the professional system of care. Both these patterns and variations may appear, at first glance, problematic to the untrained eye. Nevertheless, to develop an awareness of the complexities of psychotropic drug use implies that overall patterns of use (i.e. dependency) as well as particular, subjective experiences (i.e. individual drug-taking careers) are included within the perspective framed by the formal health care system.

As we saw in the previous chapter, the lay network played an important role in introducing users to psychotropics. Most psychotropic drug use is, however, initiated by professional help: the physician prescribes the drug and determines the dosage and duration of use. In the formal system of health care, physicians act as the main agents of introduction to, and continuation of, drug use. While physicians may appear as 'agents of dependency' – either aiding dependency or assisting in the stopping of it – users can be viewed as dependent on drug use as well as the health care system which is, in the majority of cases, the actual instigator of use.

This chapter is divided into two main sections. The first section, empirically based, is an examination of the issue of dependency, conceptualised as users become involved in the health care system. The second section focuses on theoretical concerns and contends that traditional views on drug using need to be reformulated. In turn, a view is offered on how dependency on psychotropic drugs becomes formalised through various systems of meanings and norms on both the micro and macro levels of analyses.

DEPENDENCY AND DRUG USE: EMPIRICAL CONCERNS

In the following discussion, we will examine the health status of long-term users; their views on dependency; their efforts to stop taking their drugs; their dependency on other substances; and general conclusions on dependency from the users' points of view.

The health status of long-term users

Attached to health care conceptions about long-term psychotropic drug use is the notion that this type of behaviour is not only a form of illness behaviour but that it can also take an habitual or chronic form. Nevertheless, many psychotropic drug users evaluate their health status in terms of other health measures besides the chronicity of their drug use. In this context, the majority of the drug users (70 per cent) in our empirical study reported that their health was at least average or above. However, a majority reported suffering from a chronic illness (72 per cent), and here the morbidity was almost twice as high for female (85 per cent) as for male users (44 per cent). A partial reason for this difference was the higher mean age of the female respondents. Also, in terms of the national average, the use of minor tranquillisers in Finland is twice as high among those who report a chronic illness (see Table 8.1).

Table 8.1 Distribution (%) of drug users by health status and experience of chronic illness

	Females	Males	Total
Health status			
Quite good	21	21	21
Good	4	14	8
Average	43	37	41
Bad	3	5	4
Quite bad	29	23	26
Experience of chronic illness			
Yes	85	44	72
No	15	56	28
Total (%)	100	100	100
N	57	43	100

Users' views on dependency

A majority (71 per cent) of current users wanted to stop using their psychotropic drugs. Half the current users reported that it would be difficult to stop the use, even if they wanted to. Female current users (67 per cent) reported this more frequently than male current users (42 per cent). The reasons *why users wanted to stop* using their drugs varied but a very high proportion of users (85 per cent) wanted to stop because they viewed their drug use as a dependency problem. Half the users reported that the reason *why it would be difficult for them to stop* using was related to dependency problems. A majority (59 per cent) of male users reported that reason, while females tended to split their reasons between sleeping problems (48 per cent) and dependency problems (44 per cent).

Excerpts from narratives evidenced an awareness of varying types and levels of dependency from user points of view. First, let us consider female narrators:

'I am afraid of the pills and would like to stop but cannot, so I am hooked in a way . . . I am . . . afraid of getting dependent.'

(57-year-old teacher)

'I would be happy to quit because I am afraid of their effects.'

(59-year-old dressmaker)

'I was very dependent on Halcion, even after I left work.'

(47-year-old library assistant)

'I think I am [dependent] because . . . I can be terribly anxious when I try to be without. . . . I have panic attacks; it differs from day to day when I am not taking the drug. Sometimes I feel very good when I have not taken any drugs. . . . You can say I am [dependent]. It does feel terrible, but I am . . . you get addicted to them [these drugs] to some extent. My self-confidence gets really high if I can be without them for some time.'

(33-year-old part-time cleaner)

One male user contemplates whether or not, in the context of his dependency, he may be experiencing stress:

'Yes, I am [dependent] . . . I take them [the pills] one hour before I go to sleep and they tranquillise me. I don't know maybe I feel stressed and I am a very nervous man.'

(66-year-old farmer)

Another male user, after revealing his earliest memory of the need for his drug, discussed his dependency:

'The dependency came very slowly. First, there were ten to fifteen years when I took them only when I really needed them. Perhaps it is normal with age that insomnia begins to bother you. And one gets used to them [drugs]. Then there was a physician-prescribed drug in the cabinet and I developed a habit over the years. I took them every night. The dependency was, in my opinion, mainly psychological. I did not get to sleep, I simply had to go to get something first.'

(74-year-old retired insurance director)

In recounting their experiences of dependency, female more than male users were able to retell how they actually 'felt' their dependency. While they contextualised their stories within an emotional framework, they had a sense that the drugs affected their physical well-being. Hence, they wanted to describe these effects and how and in what spaces these effects emerged. For many women, their insomnia related primarily to problems with husbands or children, although originally their drug use had begun with a physical illness. For example:

'When I go to bed in the evening, I plan that I won't take any pills and then I can't get to sleep immediately. I go to take a pill. Is that not dependency? It is like a psychological dependency. . . . I just roll about in bed and then I go to take the sleeping pill.'

(51-year-old female postal worker)

'I just felt that I couldn't fall asleep if I didn't take one – even if I didn't have to get up in the morning. It was so natural already. It was really a relief when they said that they had stopped selling it [Halcion].'

(47-year-old female library assistant)

'Basically, if I don't take [drugs] in the evening I won't get to sleep. Sometimes I fall asleep by mistake and then I am awake for several hours in the night. . . . Sometimes when I am in the country I leave them [my pills] at home. Then there is nothing I can do . . . so I am in a way psychologically hooked.'

(59-year-old female dressmaker)

'I have thought about how the dependence is psychological
... because my dose is so small. I believe that many sleeping
pill users develop a way of thinking that they cannot get to
sleep if they don't take a pill.'

(33-year-old female part-time cleaner)

One male user, also an insomnia sufferer, was unable at first to
contextualise his account of dependency. He recounted that he
was 'not dependent at all', but subsequently admitted to being
dependent when he said, 'Without my pills I would go several
nights without sleeping' (56-year-old porter).

Recognising their problems with the further stress caused
by their dependency, many long-term psychotropic drug users
believed that stopping would be beneficial to their health.
They tended to develop this belief in the context of the
possibilities available to them within the formal system of
health care – consulting their doctors.

Users' efforts to stop taking drugs

In light of the above views on dependency, some users were
active in their efforts to terminate their dependency. About
half the current users had been worried about the duration of
their drug use and discussed their desire to stop with their
doctor. This desire had received a mixed response (see Table
8.2). A third of the current users reported that their doctor had
supported their wish to stop using drugs. There was, however,
a marked gender difference in this group: male respondents
had twice as often received support from their doctor in their
desire to stop. By contrast, a third of the female current users
had been told by their doctor that there was no alternative to
their drug use; only 6 per cent of the male current users had
been told this. Furthermore, a third of both male and female
current users reported that their doctor had told them that the
drug was harmless, confirming the continuation of their drug
use. Generally, in comparison to men, women had received
less encouragement and support in their desire to stop as well
as fewer alternatives to their drug use from their doctor. This
confirms the idea of the inevitable course of women's drug
careers.

Table 8.2 Distribution (%) of current drug users by their efforts at
stopping psychotropic drug use and doctors' responses

	Females	Males	Total	
			%	N
Current users discussed stopping with doctor (N = 85)				
Yes	45	45	45	38
No	40	35	38	32
No answer	15	20	17	15
Total (%)	100	100	100	85
N	45	40		
Doctor's response to expressed desire to stop drug use (N = 38)				
Positively agreed	20	44	32	12
Said the drug was harmless	30	28	30	11
Said there was no alternative	30	6	18	7
Made no comment	10	11	10	4
Both agreed and disagreed	5	6	5	2
No answer	5	5	5	2
Total (%)	100	100	100	38
N	20	18		

Users' narratives also produced stories about whether or
not the users had ever thought of stopping. When pondering
this question, one female narrator replied in a question
directed at the listener and asked, 'Could you give up coffee?',
reflecting the impossibility of giving up for her. (Finland has a
high per capita consumption of coffee.) This woman also
disclosed that she would like to stop but felt 'addicted'. Her
doctor had told her that her drugs are not only 'not dangerous'
but also that she can 'do very well with them'. She recounted:

'I said [to my doctor] that since I am a slave to these [drugs]
I want to get rid of them but he just said that they are not
dangerous and that I could do very well with them. They
[doctors] are not at all worried about it, even if I am. If a

doctor would say that you simply do not take them any longer, it would be easy to stop. But the doctors don't really care.'

(59-year-old dressmaker)

Another female narrator told of her recent failed attempts to stop using her drugs:

'I did try to stop for a couple of nights and I didn't sleep, so I took it anyway in the early hours of the morning. I did not think before that time that I was dependent.'

(57-year-old teacher)

This user felt that her drug use was a burden, and it made her feel bad about herself. She despaired at the thought of taking these drugs, but she felt, at the same time, that she was too emotional to stop using them. In this context, she recounts some brief, successful attempts at stopping:

'Yes, I have tried to stop from time to time. Then the pressure is off and everything is fine. I feel fine. I have tried to stop, but I don't think I could now. Now, of course, in my situation no one would suggest that I don't need to take [them] but when I am so emotional – all I would do is start worrying again. I can't stop.'

One female narrator thought that it would be possible for her to stop, but she had continued support in coping with her 'stress' and depression from a professional therapist in the health care system:

'Yes, I have . . . discussed it with my therapist many times. He thinks that I should be without them, especially now when the therapy is so intense – so all my feelings could come out. He cannot otherwise repair what is there underneath. One just escapes to the medication. . . . I have been without the drugs. I do think I could stop. My confidence about it varies from day to day.

(33-year-old part-time cleaner)

When asked directly, 'Have you ever thought of stopping?' and 'Have you ever felt that you wanted to stop?', two male users revealed that thinking about stopping was a constant preoccupation with them.

Emphasising the persistent logic of the thought of stopping, the first male narrator said:

'All the time. I could, if I would sleep. If you lie awake all the time and keep turning around you will wear out your sheets. My shoulder was dislocated when I fell under a cow. It ached this morning, but I have an ointment that helps.'

(66-year-old farmer)

Echoing this theme, the second male narrator said:

'Of course, it [stopping] is always on my mind. . . . I would like to stop taking sleeping pills because soon I will get no sleep without them. . . . Yes, I think [I could stop] . . . because I do not feel that I have to take them. It is my choice and then I know that I can work the next day. Sometimes, when you wake up in the night, you get the feeling that you cannot read or listen to the radio even if you could in the evening. But you cannot when you wake up in the night. You cannot do anything. You just feel that you have to get to sleep. If I could get six-months' leave and live peacefully for that time, I am sure I would get my rhythm back. I do not doubt that at all.'

(56-year-old porter)

Users' dependency on other substances

Users also experienced dependency on other drugs, namely alcohol and nicotine. Higher percentages of male users (93 per cent and 65 per cent) in comparison with female users (39 per cent and 25 per cent) reported that they had smoked at some time during their lives and smoked at present. (See Table 8.3.) On the whole, male respondents appeared to be more frequent users of alcohol than female respondents. Twenty-nine per cent of male respondents reported that they drink beer or other alcoholic beverages daily and 24 per cent said that they do this two to three times a week, as compared to 3 per cent and 12 per cent respectively for the females. Furthermore, two-thirds of the male respondents volunteered for the study through alcohol treatment facilities. Hence, one type of chemical

Table 8.3 Distribution (%) of drug users by gender and use of tobacco and alcohol

	Females	Males	Total sample
Experienced smoking in life cycle			
Smoked	39	93	62
Never smoked	61	7	38
Current use of tobacco			
Smokes now	25	65	42
Does not smoke now	75	35	58
Frequency of alcohol use			
Daily	3	29	14
Two to three times a week	12	24	17
About once a week	9	9	9
Two to four times a month	12	26	18
Sometimes during a year	46	7	29
Never	18	5	12
Total (%)	100	100	100
N	57	43	100

dependency had most likely resulted in dependency on another substance – minor tranquillisers. Since our data were cross-sectional they did not provide information about the sequence of dependency on substances but mainly about current dependencies.

Overall conclusions about users' experiences of dependency

Our results show that current users felt it would be difficult to stop using their drugs; they wanted to stop using and saw dependency problems as being both the *cause* of difficulties in stopping and the *reason* why they wanted to stop. In short, they knew that they were dependent; they wanted to stop, they knew why and that this would be difficult, and they had discussed stopping within the formal health care setting (i.e. with their doctors).

The fact that male respondents were clearly smoking and drinking more heavily than female respondents could suggest that links between the fear of being dependent on drugs and the use of other 'addictive' substances have not yet been made either by these individuals or by their prescribers. Our results clearly show no support for a substitution hypothesis, an issue highlighted in Chapter 3, because alcohol use was mentioned by men as a reason for using psychotropic drugs, as well as an alternative substance to lessen their symptoms (as noted in the previous chapter). Whether these findings could be an artifact in the data introduced by our recruitment procedure (e.g. through alcohol clinics) or a general trend in men's patterns of use remains unclear. Nevertheless, the data do suggest a pattern of dual dependency (on psychotropics and alcohol) experienced more often by male than female respondents.

It is obvious from the above discussions on dependency that stopping use was an issue which occupied the thoughts of many users. However, in the context of the health care system, there appeared to be gendered, behavioural norms which governed doctors' views: they saw women's use of psychotropics as an inevitable course of action, while they did not view men's use in a similar way. Furthermore, doctors appeared more often than not to confirm women's rather than men's sustained use or dependency. After all, within this professional context, these drugs are perceived as an effective way of dealing with stress or anxiety. This view exists regardless of users' perceived need to stop taking drugs. The above results on users' efforts to stop their use confirm that gender and drug use are intricately linked in the professional treatment of psychiatric symptoms organised within the formal system of health care.

On a different level, both male and female users were concerned about their long-term use but women more than men had experienced feelings of guilt. In their families, women found little support for their continued use, while doctors generally saw women's use as harmless and justified. Men had a more instrumental attitude towards drug use: it maintained their working capacity. Women did not relate their drug use to maintaining a caring role, which was perceived mainly as affective rather than instrumental.

For men, their use and subsequent dependency was overt

and they legitimised their long-term use as a medical need. By contrast, the women, feeling guilty about their dependent drug use, perceived that the male attitude towards legal drugs as a form of 'pharmacological Calvinism' (Klerman 1970) was the normative pattern. 'Pharmacological Calvinism' has been defined as an attitude towards drug use which perceives it as either morally wrong or something which one has to pay for with dependence, the former perception implying a type of social transgression (an issue to be discussed below). For women, the ethic of drug use was conceptualised in Klerman's terms as, 'If a drug makes you feel good, it must be bad.' Hence, not surprisingly, many female respondents, faced with this moral imperative, tried to hide their drug use and even to begin the termination of use 'secretly'.

DEPENDENCY AND THE HEALTH CARE SYSTEM: THEORETICAL CONCERNS

We will now examine how drug dependency is organised in the context of the formal health care system by introducing four concepts: social transgressor, drug career, transitory life-cycle status and drug harm. First, we introduce the term, *social transgressor*, in light of the previous empirical discussions. Then, we examine traditional approaches to drug use and call for their reformulation. In an attempt at this reformulation, we move on to a discussion of another way of seeing the issue of psychotropic drugs: on the micro level of analysis (i.e. a focus on the discursive subject) with the aid of the concepts *drug career* and *transitory life-cycle status*, and on the macro level of analysis (i.e. a focus on the epidemiological gaze) with the related concepts of *drug harm*.

Psychotropic drug users as social transgressors

We saw from the above discussion on dependency that users themselves, particularly female users, have moralistic attitudes about their drug use. Whether this behaviour was perceived as 'bad' or somehow punishable, by becoming 'hooked' (i.e. becoming dependent), they felt, if only secretly, a sense of transgression. Their self-identities (i.e. as psychotropic drug 'addicts') were becoming their social identities. They appear as *social transgressors,* violating the social boundaries between self-control and loss of control. Additionally, they blur the boundaries between 'healthy' and 'sick' bodies. This is because they appear as 'internally polluted', what Warburton (1978) defines as 'the state when the purity of the internal environment of one's body is destroyed'. Through psychotropic drug use, their bodies are viewed as internally polluted.

From another theoretical angle, all drug users (whether legal or illegal) are not perceived as average social subjects. They are social transgressors and viewed as defying society. Therefore, they do not fit comfortably within a society based on self-control. Furthermore, they 'crave' a mind-altering substance, which is seen by others as creating chaos in sufferers' lives (George 1993). The paradox is that psychotropic drug users do appear as normal citizens and more often than not have more similarities to than differences from other non-drug using members of society (Davies 1992). Nevertheless, drug users will appear as somehow 'out of order' or beyond the boundaries of mainstream society. As a result, while all drug-taking behaviour is understood as being in need of surveillance and control, drug users emerge as transgressors.

Traditional approaches to drug use: social problems, deviance, deviant career and master status

In our attempt to reach an understanding of drug use, we must first examine the ways in which traditional approaches to the social problem of drug using, particularly illegal drug using, have been developed. We contend that this development needs to be examined further with critical, gender-sensitive eyes.

Cultural norms on drug use perpetuate the idea that, inevitably, drug problems, addiction or dependence will involve those whose behaviour is perceived by themselves or others (or both) as transgressing certain social boundaries, if not 'deviant'. As a group, sufferers become defined within the context of a social problem. This is because sufferers from 'nerves' or stress present themselves to their physicians with 'personal deviance'. They themselves may question their normality. For example, they ask themselves and/or their doctor, 'Am I normal because I suffer from "nerves" or stress?'. Like other patients who present with personal deviance, their 'illness' is likely to be interpreted by their doctor as 'deviance' (Armstrong 1989:123). Here the concepts, deviance, deviant career and master status need some attention.

From a sociological perspective, deviance is an intriguing concept which has its roots in the functionalism of the Mertonian (1957) way of thinking. For Merton, deviance was emblematic of structural strain. This notion was translated into analyses of the various legitimate as well as illegitimate means that individuals used when they confronted culturally defined goals, such as wealth and success. But Merton's conceptualisations were framed within a social consensus approach to society – an approach which upholds the status quo. His theory lacked any political (and therefore gender) aspect. For example, we have no sense, in his general conception of structural strain, of whether or not, or how, this strain was differentially experienced within structurally disadvantaged social groups (Taylor *et al.* 1973:107). Of course, women lose out in this type of deviance perspective.

Nevertheless, the definition of deviance expanded with labelling theory (Becker 1963; Lemert 1967:17). On the one hand, Becker analysed how social groups label outsiders as deviants. His analysis focused both on the micro level (in terms of the processes of deviant interactions) and the macro level (in terms of the role of moral entrepreneurs in shaping public perceptions of deviance). However, similar to Merton, Becker does not account for structural inequalities. We have little sense of the fact that conceptions of deviance as well as normality are ranked according to any deviant's structural position.

On the other hand, Lemert split deviance into two operational concepts (i.e. primary and secondary deviance). The former concept referred to deviance with marginal implications on the individual level, while the latter, secondary deviance, referred to a deeper entrenchment in deviance – one's attitude to one's self and one's social role become symbolically reorganised. But, as with Merton and Becker, Lemert lacked a structural analysis and gender was neutralised. Nevertheless, the benefits of these analyses were that the concept, deviance, previously considered marginal in sociology, was given its own analytical site, next to culture, society, social groups, etc.

An enlargement of conceptions of deviance was the term, deviant career, which was developed by Becker (1963:25–39) in an attempt to analyse how people pass through a series of stages in becoming deviant. Becker used this term, deviant career, to privilege drug taking (i.e. marijuana use) as a deviant enterprise. But, in developing this concept, Becker relied on conventional social norms of deviant and normal drug taking. As a result, his term, deviant career, shadows any understanding of drug use as a meaningful, social activity which can be performed by 'rational' human beings in pursuit of routine and order.

Another concept which Becker developed within the traditional deviant framework is 'master status'. Using 'master status' with special reference to illegal drug users (i.e. marijuana users), he borrowed this concept 'with profit' from Everett C. Hughes (1945). In Becker's view, any deviant identification becomes a 'master status', informing the advancement of a deviant career. However, there are two important reasons for re-examining this notion of master status. First, and perhaps most obvious, if a gender-sensitive perspective is aimed at, the word 'master' hints at maleness and masculinity and, therefore, hinders the development of this perspective. Second, the use of this traditional notion provides no sense of conflicting conceptions of time, local variations or differences from the user's point of view – a sense which is needed if one is to emphasise the instrumental rationality of drug users as embodied subjects. In this context, we argue that traditional approaches to drug use, framed within a social problem or deviance perspective, are limited. These approaches do not 'work' when applied to psychotropic drug use.

For example, in Chapter 2, it was demonstrated how tranquilliser use has emerged as a social problem, albeit not a gendered problem, and how this process implies the imposition of a new 'deviant' label for women. Within this limited framework, 'the awarding of deviant identity' (with the added dimension of a deviant career) permits the subject (the one awarded the deviant identity) 'little scope for negotiation or rebuttal' in society (Downes and Rock 1982:154). A concomitant effect of this process for long-term psychotropic drug users, particularly female ones, is that they are more open to

public scrutiny than ever before. A new label has been constructed – a label with implicit moral judgements. With this
development, there is a danger that the psychotropic drug
user, viewed as 'deviant', the one observed and spoken about,
and, finally, the research object, becomes silenced and unable
to speak for him- or herself as a subject.

Generally, in order to achieve a broader understanding of
psychotropic drug use, a traditional social problems or deviant
framework must be challenged. The notions provided within
these frameworks are less than adequate, particularly when
we want to look at different cultures, competing definitions of
drug use (i.e. legal versus illegal) within any given society and
gender. For example, cultures do vary in the ways they regu-
late deviant traffic moving back and forth from their outer
boundaries – a notion put forward early on by Erikson (1964).
But, along with a recognition of cultural variations, one needs
to account for the fact that psychotropic drug users move back
and forth between direct or indirect involvement in the diverse
segments of the health care system – the organisational, institutional, regulatory and financial. All these segments shape
how their transgression will be defined. There are also competing models of drug use in any given society (van de
Wijngaart 1993), making it all the more difficult to define what
offending, transgressing or 'deviant' drug use actually is.
Furthermore, when these sorts of definition of drug use do
emerge, they reveal a gendering process: there are different
definitions for men and women (Ettorre 1992).

Now that we have looked critically at the traditional
deviant or social problems framework, we want to introduce
three concepts in order to understand psychotropic drug
users: drug career, transitory life-cycle status and drug harm.
These notions operate at two levels of analysis: the micro level
and the macro level.

Drug career and psychotropic drug users

On the subjective/micro level of analysis, the concept of drug
career emerges. We define *drug career* broadly as sustained
involvement in the pursuit of drug taking within an individual's
life cycle. This is a concept borrowed and subsequently

amended from related work in the field of illegal drug use (Rosenbaum 1981; Parker *et al.* 1988; Pearson 1987; Taylor 1993; Waldorf *et al.* 1991). It is theoretically relevant for four reasons. First, drug career is a more impartial concept than the more traditional one, deviant career, and can be used as a way of bestowing non-judgemental or more neutral views of psychotropic drug use. Employing this notion allows one to examine the stake that users, as 'normal folk or ordinary citizens', have in conventional life (Waldorf *et al.* 1991).

Second, the concept, drug career, allows for acceptance of the fact that not only do drug users' lives change but also that life-cycle changes (which include drug taking) can provide meaning, motivation, security and, in some instances, status as well as personal legitimation to a number of 'normal folk' in society. Here, applying the concept, drug career, releases the possibility of recognition, if not entitlement, for previously disenfranchised groups in society: both legal and illegal drug users.

Third, in our current subject area of psychotropic drug use, the application of the concept, drug career, enables us to see the processes involved in entering, continuing and terminating use. On a related process level, using the concept drug career helps to build a picture of the advantages and disadvantages of involvement with psychotropic drugs – making important theoretical links with both the lay and professional cultures surrounding this use. In effect, discursive subjectivity and the user's point of view are emphasised.

Fourth, from the vantage point of gender, the notion of drug career is crucial. This is because it enables an active and involved picture of female psychotropic drug users to emerge, as a counterbalance to their traditional image as passive victims (Ettorre 1985) and 'more nervous or anxious than men' (Jerome 1991). Aided by this 'career' concept, any female drug user, like her male counterpart, can be characterised as a purposeful, resourceful person, responding in a deliberate way to particular sets of social circumstances (Taylor 1993). Let us now turn our attention to another notion which should be useful in developing our framework of study.

Psychotropic drug taking: a transitory life-cycle status

Clearly, within the context of traditional approaches to deviance and deviant careers, there was little room to discover how subjectivity is embodied and negotiated within the area of public health and hygiene. In an earlier context, we exposed the limitations of the concept 'master status'. Here, we contend that this concept should be replaced by a more appropriate, expansive notion: *transitory life-cycle status*. This concept refers to the notion that at certain times, over a period of time and / or in certain situations, drugs are included within a user's life cycle for a variety of reasons which may be subject to change. Privileging this notion opens up the possibility of the emergence of a more accessible, cultured individuality; upholds sufferers' experiences; and appropriates the lived life in a variety of social spaces (and not drug taking) as being the main sustenance of long-term psychotropic drug users. Here the implication is that drug taking is a sufficient but not a necessary cause of change or disruption in a user's life cycle.

For example, drug taking, with all it implies on a physical, psychological, emotional and social level, can be experienced as a major status with authoritative clout, overriding and subordinating other circumstances (e.g. one's work, family life, etc.) in one's life cycle. On the other hand, drug taking may also be experienced as a supplementary or reserve status which itself can be subordinated. If this concept is used, images and strange combinations may emerge simultaneously – elderly ladies taking high dosages of minor tranquillisers in nursing homes; 'street kids' searching for illegal street drugs; rich businessmen snorting 'coke' in office lavatories. This is not a homogeneous grouping. The picture is one of diversity, cyclicality and multiple dimensions for the drug user, restored as a subject with instrumental rationality, whether or not it appears to be expressed. To take the lead in the pursuit of the 'subject' in the field of drug studies is all about creating theoretical frameworks which reflect novel conceptualisations of both legal and illegal drug users.

DRUG HARM AND THE EPIDEMIOLOGICAL GAZE

Now let us turn our attention to wider, macro levels of concern. We will look, first, at the issue of drug harm, a concept that develops from within the epidemiological gaze and, second, at how this gaze exerts surveillance on drug users and dependency as public health issues.

Given that benzodiazepines are used also by illicit drug users who, more often than not, are poly-drug users (Seivewright *et al.* 1993; Sheehan *et al.* 1991), the use of minor tranquillisers has emerged as a visible policy concern in recent years (Ettorre 1991). Furthermore, the issue of media responses to dependence on tranquillisers has not escaped public notice (Bury and Gabe 1991). Clark (1993), a drug researcher, emphasises that there is a general social consensus about *drug harm*: all drug use causes a certain amount of personal and social harm, regardless of the legal status of the drug consumed. Unlike non-drug using members of society, drug users are viewed as socially damaged or harmed in some way by their use of drugs. In Clark's view, this consensus endures primarily because drug harm is associated with health costs (e.g. increased likelihood of accidents involving those driving or operating machinery while under the influence of drugs) and the 'environmental' effects of meeting drug users in public (i.e. similar to the nuisance effect of drunks).

While there is a general consensus surrounding the issue of drug harm, there has never been a similar consensus, either within the medical community or society in general, about how to treat emotional and social illnesses (Montagne 1991:64). Additionally, no culture has developed well-defined rituals or social sanctions to direct and control the prescribing and use of minor tranquillisers, which since their introduction have been 'doomed to controversy' (Smith 1991). Indeed, it appears that doctors may be at a 'loose end' in identifying and discussing patients' psychological and social problems. While doctors may want troubled patients to be autonomous, they may resent those who depend too much on tranquillisers. Furthermore, many doctors suspect that there is some impairment of mental functioning as a result of the use of these drugs (Horder 1991).

From the sufferer's point of view, the desired or positive consequences of drug taking (i.e. relief from stress or anxiety, uninterrupted sleep) override, at first, any conception or experience of drug harm, especially for any seasoned drug user (Tober 1989). The result is that drug taking (whether legal or illegal) tends to be mediated more by the norms, practices and circumstances of users than by the perceptions of others, including doctors – in the case of tranquilliser users.

In an earlier discussion about social transgression, the notion of drug users as being internally polluted was mentioned. Through the epidemiological gaze, the public health regime with its emphasis on 'lifestyle politics' (Armstrong 1983, 1993) can be seen as extending the idea of drug users as polluted into the realm of the body politic. Plainly, the mere existence of drug users is an encroachment on the body politic.

In the regime of public health, drug use, whether legal or illegal, is pushed into the arena of social hygiene which extends beyond the personal. This is because drug use is located within the context of wider social activities (other than drug taking), framed by the diverse segments of the health care system. For example, in the organisational and institutional segments of the health care system, drug using separates clean individuals from those who are dirty and designates which groups of drug users (i.e. depending on the drugs used) are less dirty or polluted than others. On the regulatory and financial level, drug taking involves a complex set of behavioural and cultural patterns, social interactions and political responses from governments and the pharmaceutical industry.

But this picture becomes more complex when we look at long-term psychotropic drug users. They are in a particularly invidious position – a sort of 'nowhere land' in relation to other drug users – for two reasons. First, the majority of psychotropic drug users, within the space labelled 'unhygienic', are pushed further into the repressive space of transgressors because their drug taking is viewed by others, by themselves or by both as a breach of self-control. This takes place regardless of the legitimation process undertaken by doctors who raise their illness behaviour, expressed in the form of 'nerves' or 'stress', to a socially acceptable level. Second, long-term psychotropic drug users do not wear comfortably, or identify themselves with, the label 'transgressor' or 'deviant', because their long-term drug use is not only legal but may also be symbolic of their attempt to maintain control over their lives (Helman 1981). They may experience these drugs as 'lifelines' or 'stand-bys' – needed resources (Gabe and Lipshitz-Phillips 1984) facilitating self-control, rather than as a way of abandoning self-control.

In conclusion, psychotropic drug users speak not only as gendered subjects within a variety of discourses or different fields of power/knowledge but are also spoken for within diverse segments of the health care system. Their sustained involvement in the pursuit of psychotropic drugs within their life cycles (i.e. drug careers) is embedded in a formal health care system. In this system, they act as gendered subjects, located in the institutional and discursive practices of medicine where professionals alleviate sufferers' uncomfortable moods with psychotropics.

In this chapter, we showed that, as users become part of the formal health care system, they will be affected by the medical discourse on dependency. Sufferers' awareness of their state of dependency shapes their concerns about the advantages as well as the disadvantages of drug use – which emerge both from their own and others' interrelations within the health care system. Furthermore, as these concerns are shaped, the user is caught up in a selection process whereby his or her 'current' use is defined, categorised in time and ranked within the lay and medical discourses on psychotropic drug taking. Most importantly, the sufferer is part of other systems of social ranking (e.g. age, class, race, gender, ethnicity). Hence, drug dependency stands out as an issue which appears to cut across gender barriers, while, at the same time, being firmly located within the gendered nature of drug taking.

In this sense, dependency emerges as an ever-present concern in the lives of long-term psychotropic drug users. Regardless of the fact that drug taking can be observed as a transitory life-cycle status, drug dependence is experienced subjectively as a durable, intransigent state. This is particularly true for women sufferers, who more than men are channelled into a 'dependency state' through various actors and layers: through the gendered representations of their moods in advertising; through a lay culture of stress which supports pharmacological aids to relieve uncomfortable moods; by doctors who tell them that they can use this drug because it is 'harmless'; and through a health care system whose diverse segments transform health behaviour into a drug career. Overarching these layers is an emphasis on self-control, which underpins Western society and, more importantly, the institution of gender itself which channels women into being dependent by having others dependent on them. In this context, one female narrator aptly states:

> 'My drug use goes around in a circle. I worry about my children's lives all in vain. If I could only get out of this circle, I think I could stop. But my drug use is like a mother's role. I can't get away from it. No, I can't. Do you understand?'

Hence, we know that women perceive their 'dependency state' as something to be rid of. Yet women soon become aware that this is nearly an impossibility because this state of 'chemical dependency' or 'addiction' is more often than not experienced as permanent. In this way, dependency is thought to be lodged in embodied spaces where 'addiction' waits passively to be gazed at or discovered by the doctor, significant others or by oneself. At the same time, this 'chemical dependency' is active. Dependency mobilises women's bodies to cast off uncomfortable moods; to find relief for their feminine 'nerves' and to get on the track of self-control.

In Chapter 1 we contended that gender differences in psychotropic drug use are concrete manifestations of the institution of gender in society. In the light of the framework which we have provided throughout this book, we, along with other feminist sociologists, have attempted to 'destabilise' traditional theory (Barrett and Phillips 1992) and challenge 'gender-neutral thought'. Therefore, fixing a clear 'gender-sensitive gaze' on the social mosaic of psychotropic drug taking is all about overturning traditional approaches which have the potential to categorise unfairly, if not to hurt, women.

Bibliography

Alford, R. R. (1975) *Health Care Politics: Ideological and Interest Group Barriers to Reform*, Chicago: University of Chicago Press.

Alperstein, N. M. and Peyrot, M. (1993) 'Consumer awareness of prescription drug advertising', *Journal of Advertising Research* 33, 4: 50–6.

Altekruse, J. M. and McDermott, S. W. (1987) 'Contemporary concerns of women in medicine', in S. V. Rossner (ed.) *Feminism within Science and Health Professions: Overcoming Resistance*, Oxford: Pergamon Press.

Armstrong, D. (1983) *Political Autonomy of the Body: Medical Knowledge in Britain in the Twentieth Century*, Cambridge: Cambridge University Press.

—— (1989) *An Outline of Sociology as Applied to Medicine*, Oxford: Butterworth-Heinemann.

—— (1990) 'Use of the genealogical method in the exploration of chronic illness: a research note', *Social Science and Medicine* 30, 11: 1225–7.

—— (1993) 'Public health spaces and the fabrication of identity', *Sociology* 27, 3: 393–410.

Ashton, H. and Golding, J. F. (1989) 'Tranquillisers, prevalence, predictors and possible consequences: data from a large United Kingdom survey', *British Journal of Addiction* 84: 541–6.

Avorn, J., Chen, M. and Hartley, R. (1982) 'Scientific versus commercial sources of influence on prescribing behavior of physicians', *American Journal of Medicine* 73: 4–8.

Bakka, A., Johnsen, A. and Rugstad, H. E. (1974) 'Hvem bruker angstdempende midler?', *Nordisk Medicin* 89: 89–93.

Balter, M. B., Levine, J. and Manheimer, D. I. (1974) 'Cross-national study of the extent of anti-anxiety/sedative drug use', *The New England Journal of Medicine* 290: 769–74.

Barrett, M. and Phillips, A. (1992) 'Introduction', in M. Barrett and A. Phillips (eds) *Destabilizing Theory: Contemporary Feminist Debates*, Cambridge: Polity Press.

Becker, H. (1963) *Outsiders: Studies in the Sociology of Deviance,* New York: The Free Press.

Becker, H. (1967) 'Whose side are we on?', *Social Problems* 14, 3: 239–47.

Belkaoui, A. and Belkaoui, J. (1976) 'A comparative analysis of the roles portrayed by women in print advertisements: 1958, 1970, 1972', *Journal of Marketing Research* 13, 2: 168–72.

Belknap, P. and Leonard, W. M. II (1991) 'A conceptual replication and extension of Erving Goffman's study of gender advertisements', *Sex Roles* 25: 103–18.

Bell, D. S. (1980) 'Dependence on psychotropic drugs and analgesics in men and women', in *Research Advances in Alcohol and Drug Problems,* Volume 5, New York: Plenum Press.

Bellizzi, J. A. and Milner, L. (1991) 'Gender positioning of a traditionally male-dominant product', *Journal of Advertising Research* 31, 3: 72–9.

Bepko, C. (ed.) (1991) *Feminism and Addiction,* London: The Haworth Press Ltd.

Black, D. (1988) 'Temazepam capsules', *Lancet* 1, 8594: 1114.

Blaxter, M. (1983) 'The causes of disease: women talking', *Social Science and Medicine* 17: 59–69.

Blum, R., Herxheimer, A., Stenzl, C. and Woodcock, J. (1981) 'Introduction', in R. Blum, A. Herxheimer, C. Stenzl and J. Woodcock (eds) *Pharmaceuticals and Health Policy: International Perspectives on Provision and Control of Medicines,* London: Croom Helm.

Bordo, S. (1993) 'Feminism, Foucault and the politics of the body', in C. Ramazanoglu (ed.) *Up Against Foucault,* London: Routledge.

Broom, D. and Stevens, A. (1991) 'Doubly deviant', *International Journal of Drug Policy* 2: 25–7.

Brown, P. (1989) 'The health care system: introduction', in P. Brown (ed.) *Perspectives in Medical Sociology,* Belmont, California: Wadsworth Publishing Company.

Bury, M. and Gabe, J. (1991) 'Hooked? Media responses to tranquillizer dependence', in P. Abbott and G. Payne (eds) *New Directions in the Sociology of Health,* Sussex: Falmer Press.

Butler, J. (1993) *Bodies that Matter: On the Discourse Limits of Sex,* London: Routledge.

Cafferata, G. L. and Kasper, J. (1983) *Psychotropic Drugs: Use, Expenditures and Sources of Payment,* US Department of Health and Human Services, Rockville, Md: NCHSR.

Cafferata, G. L. and Meyers, S. M. (1990) 'Pathways to psychotropic drugs: understanding the basis of gender differences', *Medical Care* 28, 4: 285–300.

Cafferata, G. L., Kasper, J. and Bernstein, A. (1983) 'Family roles, structure and stressors in relation to sex differences in obtaining psychotropic drugs', *Journal of Health and Social Behavior* 24: 132–43.

Calnan, M. (1987) *Health and Illness: The Lay Perspective,* London: Tavistock.

—— (1988) 'Lay evaluation of medicine and medical practice: report of a pilot study', *International Journal of Health Services* 18: 311–22.

Calnan, M. and Williams, S. (1992) 'Images of scientific medicine', *Sociology of Health and Illness* 14, 2: 233–54.

Cappell, H. D., Sellers, E. M. and Busto, U. (1986) 'Benzodiazepines as drugs of abuse and dependence', in *Research Advances in Alcohol and Drug Problems*, Volume 9, New York: Plenum Press.

Chanfrault-Duchet, M. (1991) 'Narrative structures, social models, and symbolic representation in the life story', in S. Berger Gluck and D. Patai (eds) *Women's Words: The Feminist Practice of Oral History*, London: Routledge.

Chapman, S. (1979) 'Advertising and psychotropic drugs: the place of myth in ideological reproduction', *Social Science and Medicine* 13A: 751–64.

Charmaz, K. (1990) '"Discovering" chronic illness: using grounded theory', *Social Science and Medicine* 30, 11: 1161–72.

Chesler, P. (1989) *Women and Madness*, 2nd edn, New York: Harcourt Brace & World.

Christie, V. (1984) 'Manns middel – og kvinnes', in *Kvinnors bruk av beroendeframkallande läkemedel: Rapport från ett nordiskt forskarmöte*, Helsinki: Nordic Council for Alcohol and Drug Research.

Clare, A. (1981) 'Psychotropic drug use in general practice in Britain', in G. Tognoni, C. Bellantuono and M. Lader (eds) *The Epidemiological Impact of Psychotropic Drugs*, Amsterdam: Elsevier.

Clark, A. (1993) 'Adding up the pros and cons', *International Journal of Drug Policy* 4, 3: 116–21.

Concar, D. (1994) 'Design your own personality', *New Scientist* 143 (12 March): 22–6.

Conrad, P. (1990) 'Qualitative research on chronic illness: a commentary on method and conceptual development', *Social Science and Medicine* 30, 11: 1257–63.

—— (1992) 'Medicalization and social control' *Annual Review of Sociology* 18: 209–32.

Cooperstock, R. (1971) 'Sex differences in the use of mood-modifying drugs: an explanatory model', *Journal of Health and Social Behavior* 12: 238–44.

Cooperstock, R. and Lennard, H. (1979) 'Some social meanings of tranquilizer use', *Sociology of Health and Illness* 1, 3: 331–47.

Cooperstock, R. and Parnell, P. (1982) 'Research on psychotropic drug use', *Social Science and Medicine* 16: 1179–96.

Courtney, A. E. and Lockeretz, S. W. (1971) 'A woman's place: analysis of the roles portrayed by women in magazine advertisements', *Journal of Marketing Research* 8, 1: 92–5.

Crawford, R. (1980) 'Healthism and the medicalization of everyday life', *International Journal of Health Services* 10: 365–88.

—— (1984) 'A cultural account of "health", control release and the social body', in J. B. McKinlay (ed.) *Issues in the Political Economy of Health Care*, London: Tavistock.

Curran, V. and Golombok, S. (1985) *Bottling It Up*, London: Faber & Faber.

Daly, M. (1990) *Gyn/Ecology: The Metaethics of Radical Feminism*, Boston: Beacon Press.

Davies, J. B. (1992) *The Myth of Addiction*, London: Harwood Academic.

Davis, D. L. and Whitten, R. G. (1988) 'Medical and popular traditions of nerves', *Social Science and Medicine* 26: 1199–208.

Dorn, N. and Murji, K. (1991) *Trafficker: Drug Markets and Law Enforcement*, London: Routledge.

Downes, D. and Rock, P. (1982) *Understanding Deviance: A Guide to the Sociology of Crime and Rule Breaking*, Oxford: Clarendon Press.

Doyal, L. with Pennell, I. (1981) *The Political Economy of Health*, London: Pluto Press.

—— (1983) 'Women, health and the sexual division of labour: a case study of the women's health movement in Britain', *International Journal of Health Services* 13, 3: 373–87.

Drummond, D. C. (1991) 'Dependence on psychoactive drugs: finding a common language', in I. B. Glass (ed.) *The International Handbook of Addiction Behaviour*, London: Tavistock/Routledge.

DuPont, R. L. (1990) 'Benzodiazepines and chemical dependence: guidelines for clinicians', *Substance Abuse* 11, 4: 232–6.

Dworkin, A. (1983) *Right-wing Women: The Politics of Domesticated Females*, London: Women's Press.

Erikson, K. (1964) 'Notes on the sociology of deviance', in H. Becker (ed.) *The Other Side*, New York: The Free Press.

Ettorre, B. (1985) 'Psychotropics, passivity and the pharmaceutical industry', in A. Hensman, R. Lewis and T. Maylon (eds) *The Big Deal: The Politics of the Illicit Drugs Business*, London: Pluto Press.

Ettorre, B. (1991) 'Developments in public policy in respect of tranquilizers: a case study of Britain', *International Journal of the Addictions* 26, 11: 1233–45.

Ettorre, E. M. (1986) 'Self-help groups as an alternative to benzodiazepine use', in J. Gabe and P. Williams (eds) *Tranquillisers: Social, Psychological and Clinical Perspectives*, London: Tavistock.

Ettorre, E. (1992) *Women and Substance Use*, London: Macmillan Press.

Evans, M. (1993) 'Reading lives: how the personal might be social', *Sociology* 27, 1: 5–13.

Everett, S.E. (1991) 'Lay audience response to prescription drug advertising', *Journal of Advertising Research* 31, 2: 43–9.

Fee, E. (1983) 'Women and health care: the comparison of theories', in E. Fee (ed.) *Women and Health: The Politics of Sex in Medicine*, New York: Baywood Publishing Company.

Ferrence, R. G. (1980) 'Sex differences in the prevalence of problem drinking', in *Research Advances in Alcohol and Drug Problems*, Volume 5, New York: Plenum Press.

Ferrence, R. G. and Whitehead, P. C. (1980) 'Sex differences in psychoactive drug use: recent epidemiology', in *Research Advances in Alcohol and Drug Problems*, Volume 5, New York: Plenum Press.

Figlio, K. (1987) 'The lost subject of medical sociology', in G. Scambler (ed.) *Sociological Theory and Medical Sociology*, London: Tavistock.

Fisher, S. (1986) *In the Patient's Best Interest: Women and the Politics of Medical Decisions*, New Brunswick, New Jersey: Rutgers University Press.

Ford, J. D. and LaTour, M. S. (1993) 'Differing reactions to female role portrayals in advertising', *Journal of Advertising Research* 33, 5: 43–52.

Foucault, M. (1975) *The Birth of the Clinic: An Archeology of Medical Perception*, New York: Vintage Press.

Fox, N. J. (1993) *Postmodernism, Sociology and Health*, Buckingham: Open University Press.

Frank, A. (1990) 'Bringing bodies back: a decade review', *Theory, Culture and Society* 7: 131–62.

Freidson, E. (1960) 'Client control and medical practice', *American Journal of Sociology* 65: 374–82.

Gabe, J. (1991a) 'Personal troubles and public issues: the sociology of long-term tranquilliser use', in J. Gabe (ed.) *Understanding Tranquilliser Use: The Role of the Social Sciences*, London: Tavistock/Routledge.

—— (ed.) (1991b) *Understanding Tranquilliser Use: The Role of the Social Sciences*, London: Tavistock/Routledge.

—— and Bury, M. (1988) 'Tranquillisers as a social problem', *The Sociological Review* 36, 2: 320–52.

—— and Bury, M. (1991a) 'Drug use and dependence as a social problem: sociological approaches', in I. B. Glass (ed.) *The Inter- national Handbook of Addiction Behaviour*, London: Tavistock/Routledge.

—— and Bury, M. (1991b) 'Tranquillisers and health care in crisis', *Social Science and Medicine* 32, 4: 449–54.

Gabe, J. and Lipshitz-Phillips, S. (1984) 'Tranquillisers as social control?', *Sociological Review* 32, 3: 524–46.

Gabe, J. and Thorogood, N. (1986) 'Prescribed drug use and the management of everyday life: the experiences of black and white working-class women', *Sociological Review* 34: 737–72.

Gabe, J., Gustafsson, U. and M. Bury (1991) 'Mediating illness: newspaper coverage of tranquilliser dependence', *Sociology of Health and Illness* 13, 4: 332–53.

Gamman, L. and Marshment, M. (1988) *Female Gaze: Women as Viewers of Popular Culture*, London: The Women's Press.

George, M. (1993) 'The role of personal rules and accepted beliefs in the self-regulation of drug taking', *International Journal of Drug Policy* 4, 1: 32–5.

Gerhardt, U. (1989) *Ideas About Illness: An Intellectual and Political History of Medical Sociology*, London: Macmillan.

Giddens, A. (1991) *The Transformation of Intimacy: Sexuality, Love and Eroticism in Modern Societies*, Cambridge: Polity Press.

Glaser, B. G. and Strauss, A. L. (1967) *The Discovery of Grounded Theory*, London: Weidenfeld & Nicolson.

Goffman, E. (1961) *Asylums*, New York: Anchor.

Goffman, E. (1976) *Gender Advertisements*, Cambridge, MA: Harvard University Press.

Goldman, R. and Montagne, M. (1986) 'Marketing "mind mechanics": decoding antidepressant drug advertisements', *Social Science and Medicine* 22: 1047–58.

Gossop, M. (1988) *Living with Drugs*, 2nd edn, London: Temple Smith.

Gottlieb, M. (1975) 'Pills: pros and cons or medications for school problems', *Acta Symbolica* 6, 3: 35–65.

Graham, H. (1983) 'Caring: a labour of love', in J. Finch and D. Groves (eds) *A Labour of Love: Women, Work and Caring*, London: Routledge.

—— (1984) *Women, Health and the Family*, Brighton: Wheatsheaf.

—— (1990) 'Behaving well: women's health behaviour in context', in H. Roberts (ed.) *Women's Health Counts*, London: Routledge.

Graham, H. and Oakley, A. (1991) 'Competing ideologies of reproduction: medical and maternal perspectives on pregnancy', in C. Currer and M. Stacey (eds) *Concepts of Health and Illness: A Comparative Perspective*, Oxford: Berg.

Gudex, C. (1991) 'Adverse effects of benzodiazepines', *Social Science and Medicine* 33, 5: 587–96.

Gusfield, J. (1963) *Symbolic Crusade: Status, Politics and the American Temperance Movement*, Urbana: University of Illinois Press.

Haddon, C. (1984) *Women and Tranquillizers*, London: Sheldon Press.

Hafner, S. (1992) *Nice Girls Don't Drink: Stories of Recovery*, New York: Bergin & Garvey.

Hamlin, M. and Hammersley, D. (1989a) *The Withdraw Pack*, Birmingham: Withdraw Workshops.

—— (1989b) *The Benzodiazepine Manual: A Professional Guide to Withdrawal*, Birmingham: Withdraw Workshops.

—— (1990) 'Managing benzodiazepine withdrawal', in G. Bennett (ed.) *Treating Drug Abusers*, London: Routledge.

Hansen, E. H. (1989) 'How widely do women and men differ in their use of psychotropic drugs?: a review of Danish studies', *Journal of Social and Administrative Pharmacy* 6, 4: 165–83.

Hansen, E. H. and Gyldmark, M. (1990) *Psykofarmaka forbruget: fordeling og udvikling*, Kobenhavn: Sundhedsstyrelsen / Forebyggelse og hygiejne 12.

Harding, S. (1991) *Whose Science? Whose Knowledge?: Thinking from Women's Lives*, Ithaca: Cornell University Press.

Hatfield, B. (1987) 'Groupwork with users of minor tranquillisers', *Practice* 1: 53–62.

Hawkins, J. W. and Aber, C. S. (1988) 'The content of advertisements in medical journals: distorting the image of women', *Women and Health* 14: 43–59.

—— (1993) 'Women in advertisements in medical journals', *Sex Roles* 28, 3/4: 233–42.

Heath, S. (1987) 'Male feminism', in A. Jardine and P. Smith (eds) *Men in Feminism*, London: Methuen.

Helman, C. G. (1981) '"Tonic", "fuel" and "food": social and symbolic aspects of the long-term use of psychotropic drugs', *Social Science and Medicine* 15B: 521–33.

Hemminki, E. (1975) 'Review of literature on factors affecting drug prescribing', *Social Science and Medicine* 9: 111–15.

Henderson, S. (1993) 'Fun, *frisson* and fashion', *International Journal of Drug Policy* 4, 3: 122–9.

Herxheimer, A. and Stimson, G. (1981) 'The use of medicines for illness', in R. Blum, A. Herxheimer, C. Stenzl and J. Woodock (eds) *Pharmaceuticals and Health Policy: International Perspectives on Provision and Control of Medicines*, London: Croom Helm.

Hohmann, A. A. (1989) 'Gender bias in psychotropic drug prescribing in primary care', *Medical Care* 27: 478–90.

Holland, J., Ramazanoglu, C., Sharpe, S. and Thomas, R. (1993) 'Power and desire: the embodiment of female sexuality', *Feminist Review* 46: 21–38.

Horder, J. (1991) 'Long-term tranquilliser use: a general practitioner's view', in J. Gabe (ed.) *Understanding Tranquilliser Use: The Role of the Social Sciences*, London: Tavistock/Routledge.

Horowitz, A. (1977) 'The pathways into psychiatric treatment: some differences between men and women', *Journal of Health and Social Behavior* 18: 169–78.

Hser, Y. Anglin, M. D. and McGlothlin, W. (1987) 'Sex differences in addict careers: I. Initiation of use', *American Journal of Drug and Alcohol Abuse* 13, 1 and 2: 33–57.

Hughes, E. C. (1945) 'Dilemmas and contradictions of status', *American Journal of Sociology* L (March): 353–9.

Hägglund, U. (1991) 'Kvinnor i läkemedelsreklam: en studie av psykofarmakareklamen i nordiska läkartidskrifter', in U. Hägglund and E. Riska (eds) *Kvinnors hälsa och ohälsa*, Åbo / Turku: Institute of Women's Studies, Åbo Akademy University.

Hägglund, U. and Riska, E. (1993) 'Advertisements for tranquillizers and hypnotics-sedatives in Denmark, Finland, and Sweden', in E. Riska, E. Kuhlhorn, S. Nordlund and K. T. Skinhøj (eds) *Minor Tranquillizers in the Nordic Countries*, Helsinki: Nordic Council for Alcohol and Drug Research.

Isacson, D. and Haglund, B. (1988) 'Psychotropic drug use in a Swedish community: the importance of demographic and socioeconomic factors', *Social Science and Medicine* 26: 477–83.

Isacson, D. Bingefors, K., Wennberg, M. and Dahlström M. (1993) 'Factors associated with high-quantity prescriptions of benzodiazepines in Sweden', *Social Science and Medicine* 36: 343–51.

Iyer, E. and Debevec, K. (1986) 'Gender stereotyping of products: are products like people?', in N. K. Maholtra and J. M. Hawes (eds) *Developments in Marketing Science*, Atlanta: Academy of Marketing Science.

Jartsell, B. and Nordegren, T. (1976) *Ångest för miljoner: Läkemedelsmissbruk i Sverige*, Ystad: Raben & Sjögren.

Jerome, J. with Bilgori, L. (1991) *The Lost Years: Tranquillisers and After*, London: Virgin Publishing.

Johnson, K. and Dawson, L. (1990) 'Women's health as multidisciplinary specialty', *Journal of American Women's Medical Association*, 45: 225–6.

Järvinen, M. and H. Olafsdottir (1989) 'Drinking patterns in the Nordic countries', in E. Haavio-Mannila (ed.) *Women, Alcohol and Drugs in the Nordic Countries*, Helsinki: Nordic Council for Alcohol and Drug Research.

Kalant, O. J. (1980) 'Sex differences in alcohol and drug problems – highlights', in *Research Advances in Alcohol and Drug Problems*, Volume 5, New York: Plenum Press.

Katz, A. (1981) 'Self-help and mutual aid: an emerging movement', *Annual Review of Sociology* 7: 129–55.

Klassen, M. L., Jasper, C. R. and Schwartz, A. M. (1993) 'Men and women: images of their relationships in magazine advertisements', *Journal of Advertising Research* 33, 2: 30–9.

Kleinman, A. (1988) *The Illness Narratives: Suffering, Healing and the Human Condition*, New York: Basic Books.

Klerman, G. L. (1970) 'Drugs and social values', *International Journal of the Addictions* 5: 313–19.

Koumjian, K. (1981) 'The use of Valium as a form of social control', *Social Science and Medicine* 15: 240–8.

Kramer, P. (1993) *Listening to Prozac*, New York: Penguin Books, USA, Inc.

Krupka, L. R. and Vener, A. (1985) 'Prescription drug advertising: trends and implications', *Social Science and Medicine* 20: 191–7.

Lader, M. (1978) 'Benzodiazepines – the opium of the masses', *Neuroscience* 3: 159–65.

—— (1991) 'Benzodiazepine withdrawal', in I. B. Glass (ed.) *The International Handbook of Addiction Behaviour*, London: Tavistock/ Routledge.

Lakoff, G. and Johnson, M. (1980) *Metaphors We Live By*, Chicago: University of Chicago Press.

Law, S. M. (1985) 'Culturally interpreted symptoms or culture-bound syndromes', *Social Science and Medicine* 21: 187–96.

Leigh, T. W., Rethans, A. J. and Whitney, R. (1987) 'Role portrayals of women in advertising: cognitive responses and advertising effectiveness', *Journal of Advertising Research* 27, 5: 54–63.

Leiss, W., Kline, S. and Jhally, S. (1986) *Social Communication in Advertising: Persons, Products and Images of Well-Being*, Toronto: Methuen.

Lemert, E. M. (1967) *Human Deviance, Social Problems and Social Control*, Englewood Cliffs, N.J.: Prentice-Hall.

Leppard, W., Ogletree, S. M. and Wallen, E. (1993) 'Gender stereotyping in medical advertising: much ado about something', *Sex Roles* 29: 822–38.

Levine, H. G. (1980) 'Temperance and women in the 19th century United States', in *Research Advances in Alcohol and Drug Problems*, Volume 5, New York: Plenum Press.

Lexchin, J. (1987) 'Pharmaceutical promotion in Canada: convince them or confuse them', *International Journal of Health Services* 17: 77–89.

—— (1989) 'Doctors and detailers: therapeutic education or pharmaceutical promotion', *International Journal of Health Services* 19: 663–79.

—— (1994) 'Canadian marketing codes: how well are they controlling pharmaceutical promotion?', *International Journal of Health Services* 24: 91–104.

Linn, L. S. (1971) 'Physician characteristics and attitudes toward legitimate use of psychotherapeutic drugs', *Journal of Health and Social Behavior* 12: 132–40.

Linn, L. S. and Davis, M. S. (1971) 'The use of psychotherapeutic drugs by middle-aged women', *Journal of Health and Social Behavior* 12: 331–40.

Lorber, J. (1975) 'Good patients and problem patients: conformity and deviance in general hospitals', *Journal of Health and Social Behavior* 16: 213–25.

—— (1994) *Paradoxes of Gender*, New Haven: Yale University Press.

MacGregor, S., Ettorre, B., Coomber, R. and Crosier, A. (1992) 'Paradigms and practice: changes in drug service ideology since the central funding initiative', *International Journal on Drugs Policy* 3, 1: 16–27.

McKinlay, J. B. (1973) 'Social networks, lay consultation and help-seeking behavior', *Social Forces* 51: 275–92.

Mant, A. and Darroch, D. B. (1975) 'Media images and medical images', *Social Science and Medicine* 9: 613–18.

Marks, J. (1982) 'The benzodiazepines – for good or evil', *International Pharmacopsychiatry* 17: 342–58.

—— (1983) 'The benzodiazepines: an international perspective', *Journal of Psychoactive Drugs* 15, 1–2: 137–49.

Martin, E. (1988) 'Medical metaphors of women's bodies: menstruation and menopause', *International Journal of Health Services* 18, 2: 237–54.

—— (1989) *The Woman in the Body: A Cultural Analysis of Reproduction*, Boston: Beacon Press.

—— (1991) 'The egg and the sperm: how science has constructed a romance based on stereotypical male–female roles', *Signs* 16: 485–501.

Maynard, M. (1990) 'The re-shaping of sociology: trends in the study of gender', *Sociology* 24: 269–90.

Medawar, C. (1992) *Power and Dependence: Social Audit on the Safety of Medicines*, Bath: Bath Press.

Mellow, G. O. (1989) 'Sustaining our organizations: feminist health activism in an age of technology', in K. Strother Rarcliff (ed.) *Health Technology: Feminist Perspectives*, Ann Arbor: University of Michigan Press.

Melville, J. (1984) *The Tranquilliser Trap and How to Get Out of It*, London: Fontana Paperbacks.

Merton, R. K. (1957) *Social Theory and Social Structure*, New York: The Free Press.

Metha, K. K., Sorofman, B. A. and Rowland, C. R. (1989) 'Prescription drug advertising trends: a study of oral hypoglycemics', *Social Science and Medicine* 29: 853–7.

Miles, A. (1988) *Women and Mental Health*, Brighton: Wheatsheaf Books.

Miles, A. (1991) *Women, Health and Medicine*, Milton Keynes: Open University Press.

Mills, C. W. (1959) *The Sociological Imagination*, Harmondsworth: Penguin Books Ltd.

Mondanaro, J. (1989) *Chemically Dependent Women: Assessment and Treatment*, Lexington, MA: Lexington Books.

Montagne, M. (1988) 'The metaphorical nature of drugs and drug taking', *Social Science and Medicine* 26, 4: 417–24.

—— (1991) 'The culture of long-term tranquilliser users', in J. Gabe (ed.) *Understanding Tranquilliser Use: The Role of the Social Sciences*, London: Tavistock/Routledge.

Mullen, K. (1994) 'Control and responsibility: moral and religious issues in lay health accounts', *Sociological Review* 42, 3: 414–37.

Murray, J. (1981) 'Long-term psychotropic drug taking and the process of withdrawal', *Psychological Medicine* 11: 853–8.

Murray, J., Williams, P. and Clare, A. (1982) 'Health and social characteristics of long-term psychotropic drug takers', *Social Science and Medicine* 16: 1595–8.

Nathanson, C. A. (1975) 'Illness and the feminine role: a theoretical review', *Social Science and Medicine* 9, 2: 57–62.

—— (1977) 'Sex, illness and medical care: a review of data, theory and method', *Social Science and Medicine* 11: 13–25.

Nations, M. K., Camino, L. A. and Walker, F. B. (1988) 'Nerves: folk idiom for anxiety and depression?', *Social Science and Medicine* 26: 1245–59.

Navarro, V. (1976) *Medicine under Capitalism*, New York: Prodist.

Neill, J. R. (1989) 'A social history of psychotropic drug advertisements', *Social Science and Medicine* 28: 333–8.

Olfson, M. and Klerman, G. L. (1993) 'Trends in the prescriptions of psychotropic medications', *Medical Care* 31: 559–64.

Orbach, S. (1978) *Fat is a Feminist Issue*, London: Paddington Press.

O'Sullivan, S. (1987) *Women's Health: A 'Spare Rib' Reader*, London: Pandora.

Owen, R. T. and Tyrer, P. (1983) 'Benzodiazepine dependence', *Drugs* 25: 385–98.

Parker, H., Bakx, K. and Newcombe, R. (1988) *Living with Heroin*, Milton Keynes: Open University Press.

Parish, P. A. (1971) 'The prescribing of psychotropic drugs in general practice', *Journal of the Royal College of General Practitioners* 21: Supplement 4.

Parry, H. J. (1968) 'Use of psychotropic drugs by U.S. adults', *Public Health Reports* 83, 10: 799–810.

Parry, H. J., Balter, M. B., Mellinger, G. D., Cisin, I. H., Manheimer, D.

I. (1973) 'National patterns of psychotherapeutic drug use, *Archives of General Psychiatry* 28: 769–83.

Parry, H. J., Cisin, I. H., Balter, M. B., Mellinger, G. D. and Manheimer, D. I. (1974) 'Increasing alcohol intake as a coping mechanism for psychic distress', in R. Cooperstock (ed.) *Social Aspects of Medical Use of Psychotropic Drugs*, Toronto: Alcoholism and Drug Addiction Research Foundation of Ontario.

Parsons, T. (1942) 'Age and sex in the social structure of the United States', *American Sociological Review* 7: 604–16.

—— (1951) *The Social System*, New York: The Free Press.

—— (1958) 'Definitions of health and illness in the light of American values and social structure', in E. Gartly Jaco (ed.) *Patients, Physicians and Illness*, Glencoe, Illinois: Free Press.

Pearson, G. (1987) *The New Heroin Users*, Oxford: Basil Blackwell.

Peay, M. Y. and Peay, E. R. (1988) 'The role of commercial sources in the adoption of a new drug', *Social Science and Medicine* 26: 1183–9.

—— (1990) 'Patterns of preference for information sources in the adoption of new drugs by specialists', *Social Science and Medicine* 31: 467–76.

Petursson, H. and Lader, M. (1981) 'Benzodiazepine dependence', *British Journal of Addiction* 76: 133–45.

Pflanz, M., Basler, H. D. and Schwoon, D. (1977) 'Use of tranquilizing drugs by a middle-aged population in a West German city', *Journal of Health and Social Behavior* 18: 194–205.

Plummer, K. (1983) *Documents of Life: An Introduction to the Problems and Literature of a Humanistic Method*, London: George Allen & Unwin.

Pohls, M. (1990) 'Women's work in Finland 1870–1940', in M. Manninen and P. Setälä (eds) *The Lady with the Bow*, Helsinki: Otava Publishing Company.

Porpora, D. V. (1986) 'Physicians' prescriptions of tranquilizers and tranquilizer abuse', *International Journal of the Addictions* 21: 559–77.

Prakash, V. (1992) 'Sex roles and advertising preferences', *Journal of Advertising Research* 32, 3: 43–51.

Prather, J. E. (1991) 'De-coding advertising: the role of communication studies in explaining the popularity of minor tranquillisers', in J. Gabe (ed.) *Understanding Tranquilliser Use: The Role of the Social Sciences*, London: Tavistock/Routledge.

Prather, J. E. and Fidell, L. S. (1975) 'Sex differences in the content and style of medical advertisements', *Social Science and Medicine* 9: 23–6.

Pugliesi, K. (1992) 'Women and mental health: two traditions of feminist research', *Women and Health* 19, 2/3: 43–68.

Rantalaiho, L. (1993) 'Gender system of the Finnish society', in L. Rantalaiho (ed.) *Social Changes and the Status of Women: The Experience of Finland and the USSR*, Tampere: University of Tampere.

Raynes, N. V. (1979) 'Factors affecting the prescribing of psychotropic drugs in general practice', *Psychological Medicine* 9: 671–9.

Riessman, C. K. (1992) 'Women and medicalization: a new

perspective', in G. Kirkup and L. Smith Keller (eds) *Inventing Women: Science, Technology and Gender*, Cambridge: Polity Press.

Riska, E. and Hägglund, U. (1991) 'Advertising for psychotropic drugs in the Nordic countries: metaphors, gender and life situations', *Social Science and Medicine* 32: 564–71.

Riska, E. and Klaukka, T. (1984) 'Use of psychotropics in Finland', *Social Science and Medicine* 19: 983–9.

Riska, E. and Wegar, K. (1995) 'The medical profession in the Nordic countries: medical uncertainty and gender-based work', in T. Johnson, G. Larkin and M. Saks (eds) *Health Professions and the State in Europe*, London: Routledge.

Riska, E., Klaukka, T., Nordlund, S. and Skinhøj, K. T. (1993) 'Use of minor tranquillizers', in E. Riska, E. Kuhlhorn, S. Nordlund and K. T. Skinhøj (eds) *Minor Tranquillizers in the Nordic Countries*, Helsinki: Nordic Council for Alcohol and Drug Research.

Roberts, H. (1991a) *Women's Health Counts*, London: Routledge.

—— (1991b) *Women's Health Matters*, London: Routledge.

Robinson, I. (1990) 'Personal narratives, social careers and medical discourses: analysing life trajectories in autobiographies of people with multiple sclerosis', *Social Science and Medicine* 30, 11: 1173–86.

Rosenau, P. M. (1992) *Post-modernism and the Social Sciences: Insights, Inroads and Intrusions*, Princeton: Princeton University Press.

Rosenbaum, M. (1981) *Women on Heroin*, New Brunswick, NJ: Rutgers University Press.

Rudman, W. J. and Hagiwara, A. F. (1992) 'Sexual exploitation in advertising health and wellness products', *Women and Health* 18: 77–89.

Rudman, W. J. and Verdi, P. (1993) 'Exploitation: comparing sexual and violent imagery of females and males in advertising', *Women and Health* 20: 1–14.

Ruzek, S. (1976) *The Women's Health Movement*, New York: Praeger.

Salmose, K. (1989) 'Women's use of alcohol in an historical perspective', in E. Haavio-Mannila (ed.) *Women, Alcohol and Drugs in the Nordic Countries*, Helsinki: Nordic Council for Alcohol and Drug Research.

Sargent, M. (1992) *Women, Drugs and Policy in Sydney, London and Amsterdam*, Aldershot: Avebury Press.

Scambler, A., Scambler, G. and Craig, D. (1981) 'Kinship and friendship networks and women's demand for primary care', *Journal of the Royal College of General Practitioners* 26: 746–50.

Scheff, T. (1966) *Being Mentally Ill*, Chicago: Aldine Publishing Co.

Seidenberg, R. (1971) 'Drug advertising and perception of mental illness', *Mental Hygiene* 55: 21–31.

Seivewright, N., Donmall, M. and Daly, C. (1993) 'Benzodiazepines in the illicit drugs scene: the UK picture and some treatment dilemmas', *International Journal of Drug Policy* 4, 1: 41–8.

Sheehan, M. F., Sheehan, D. V., Torres, A. and Coppola, E. F. (1991) 'Snorting benzodiazepines', *American Journal of Drug and Alcohol Abuse* 17: 457–68.

Shilling, C. (1993) *The Body and Social Theory*, London: Sage Publications.

Showalter, E. (1985) *The Female Malady: Women, Madness and English Culture, 1830–1980*, London: Virago Press.

Skirrow, J. (1993) 'Politics and the war on drugs', *International Journal of Drug Policy* 4, 4: 194–201.

Silverman, D. (1987) *Communication and Medical Practice: Social Relations in the Clinic*, London: Sage Publications.

Smart, C. (1984) 'Social policy and drug addiction', *British Journal of Addiction* 79, 1: 31–9.

Smith, D. (1990) *Texts, Facts and Femininity: Exploring the Relations of Ruling*, London: Routledge.

Smith, M. C. (1991) *A Social History of the Minor Tranquilizers: The Quest for Small Comfort in the Age of Anxiety*, London: Pharmaceutical Products Press.

Spitzer, S. (1975) 'Toward a Marxian theory of deviance', *Social Problems* 22: 638–51.

Stacey, M. (1988) *The Sociology of Health and Healing*, London: Unwin Hyman.

Stanley, L. (ed.) (1990) *Feminist Praxis*, London: Routledge.

Sterling, S. (1989) 'Benzodiazepines', *SCODA Newsletter*, July–August, 5–7.

Suffet, F. and Brotman, R. (1976) 'Female drug use: some observations', *International Journal of the Addictions* 11: 19–33.

Sullivan, G. L. and O'Connor, P. J. (1988) 'Women's role portrayals in magazine advertising 1958–1983', *Sex Roles* 18: 181–8.

Summers, R. S., Schutte, A. and Summers, B. (1990) 'Benzodiazepine use in a small community hospital', *South African Medical Journal* 78, 15: 721–5.

Swingewood, A. (1993) *A Short History of Sociological Thought*, 2nd edn, New York: St Martin's Press.

Taylor, A. (1993) *Women Drug Users: An Ethnography of a Female Injecting Community*, Oxford: Clarendon Press.

Taylor, I., Walton, P. and Young, J. (1973) *The New Criminology: For a Social Theory of Deviance*, London: Routledge & Kegan Paul.

Theriot, N. M. (1993) 'Women's voices in nineteenth-century medical discourse: a step toward deconstructing science', *Signs* 19: 1–31.

Thompson, E. L. (1979) 'Sexual bias in drug advertisements', *Social Science and Medicine* 13A: 187–91.

Tober, G. (1989) 'Changing conceptions of the nature of drug abuse', in G. Bennett (ed.) *Treating Drug Abusers*, London: Routledge.

Tognoni, G., Bellantuono, C. and Lader, M. (eds) (1981) *The Epidemiological Impact of Psychotropic Drugs*, Amsterdam: Elsevier.

Trickett, S. (1991) *Coming Off Tranquillisers and Sleeping Pills: A Withdrawal Plan that Really Works*, London: Thorsons Publishing Group.

Turner, B. (1984) *The Body and Society: Explorations in Social Theory*, Oxford: Basil Blackwell.

—— (1987) *Medical Power and Social Knowledge*, London: Sage Publications.

—— (1992) *Regulating Bodies: Essays in Medical Sociology*, London: Routledge.

Tyrer, P. (1974) 'The benzodiazepine bonanza', *Lancet* 2, 7882: 709–10.

van de Wijngaart, G. (1993) 'Competing perspectives on drug use', *International Journal of Drug Policy* 4, 4: 202–9.

Verbrugge, L. M. (1985) 'Gender and health: an update on hypotheses and evidence', *Journal of Health and Social Behavior* 26, 3: 156–82.

—— (1989) 'The twain meet: empirical explanation of sex differences in health and mortality', *Journal of Health and Social Behavior* 30, 3: 282–304.

Waitzkin, H. (1991) *The Politics of Medical Encounters*, New Haven: Yale University Press.

Walby, S. (1990) *Theorizing Patriarchy*, Oxford: Basil Blackwell.

Waldorf, D., Reinarman, C. and Murphy, S. (1991) *Cocaine Changes: The Experience of Using and Quitting*, Philadelphia: Temple University Press.

Waldron, I. (1977) 'Increased prescribing of Valium, Librium, and other drugs – an example of the influence of economic and social factors on the practice of medicine', *International Journal of Health Services* 7, 1: 37–62.

Walton, H. (1980) 'Ad recognition and prescribing by physicians', *Journal of Advertising Research* 20, 3: 39–48.

Warburton, D. M. (1978) 'Internal pollution', *Journal of Biosocial Science* 10: 309–19.

Wells, K. B., Kamberg, C., Brook, R., Camp, P. and Rogers, W. (1985) 'Health status, sociodemographic factors, and the use of prescribed psychotropic drugs', *Medical Care* 23: 1295–306.

Williams, G. (1984) 'The genesis of chronic illness: narrative reconstruction', *Sociology of Health and Illness* 6, 2: 175–200.

Williams, P. and Bellantuono, C. (1991) 'Long-term tranquilliser use: the contribution of epidemiology', in J. Gabe (ed.) *Understanding Tranquilliser Use: The Role of the Social Sciences*, London: Tavistock/Routledge.

Williams, R. (1993) 'Advertising: the magic system', in S. During (ed.) *The Cultural Studies Reader*, London: Routledge.

Women's National Commission (1988) *Stress and Addiction amongst Women*, London: Cabinet Office.

Woodcock, J. (1970) 'Long-term consumers of psychotropic drugs', in M. Balint, J. Hunt, D. Joyce, M. Marinker and J. Woodcock (eds) *Treatment or Diagnosis: A Study of Repeat Prescriptions in General Practice*, London: Tavistock.

Young, A. (1980) 'The discourse on stress and the reproduction of conventional knowledge', *Social Science and Medicine* 14B: 133–46.

Zola, I. (1972) 'Medicine as an institution of social control', *Sociological Review* 20: 487–504.

—— (1991) 'Bringing our bodies and ourselves back in: reflections on a past, present and future "medical sociology"', *Journal of Health and Social Behavior* 32, 1: 1–6.

Name index

Subject index

T - #0180 - 071024 - C0 - 216/138/10 - PB - 9780415082143 - Gloss Lamination